21-Day Ketogenic Diet Weight Loss Challenge

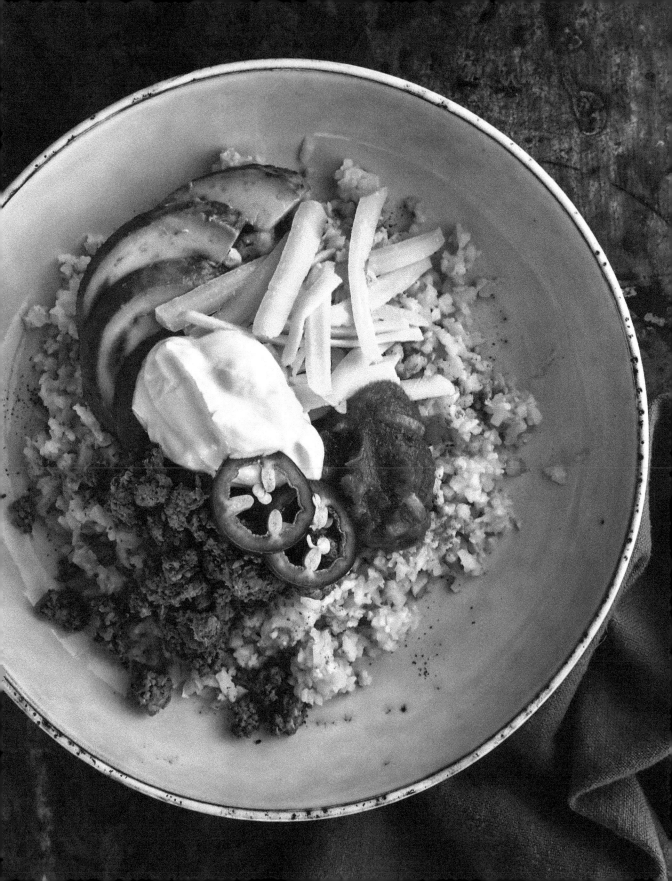

21-DAY

KETOGENIC DIET
WEIGHT LOSS
CHALLENGE

Recipes and Workouts
for a Slimmer, Healthier You

RACHEL GREGORY, MS, CNS

WITH AMANDA C. HUGHES

ROCKRIDGE
PRESS

This book is dedicated to all those ready
to embark on this challenge—
it's time to take control of your health
and become the best version of yourself!

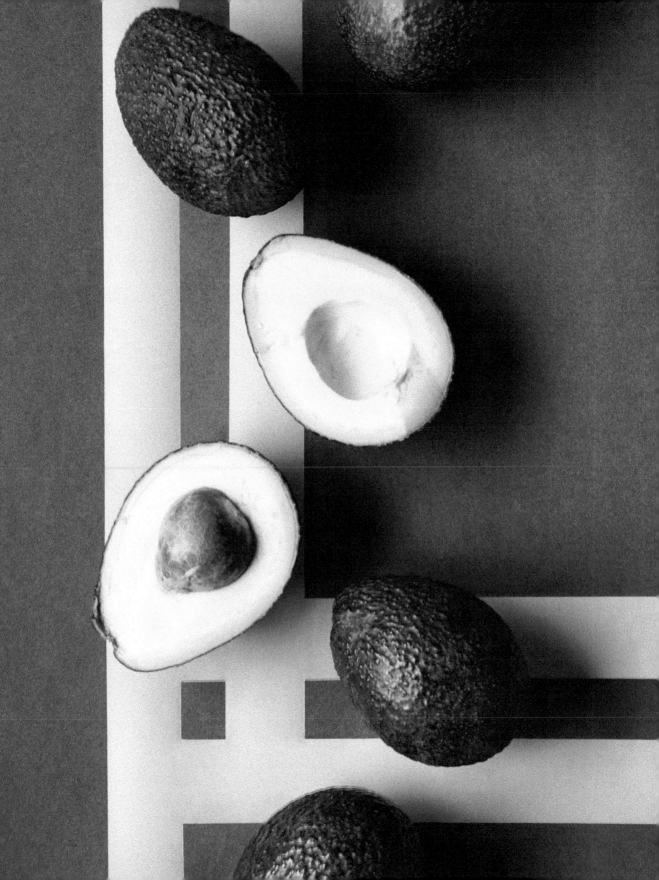

CONTENTS

A NOTE FROM Rachel

Welcome to The 21-Day Keto Challenge! The ketogenic diet is more than just a "diet." It is an extremely powerful and sustainable lifestyle that allows you to heal your body and work toward optimal health and wellness. It is a journey that requires commitment to learning, being open to change, and exploring new and unconventional ways of thinking and living. It begins as a challenge and turns into a normal way of life. When done correctly, a ketogenic protocol can contribute to easy and sustained weight loss and an overall increase in quality of life.

This 21-Day Keto Challenge targets weight loss while also taking a holistic approach to achieving lasting results by making changes to not only your diet, but also other key areas including sleep, mind-set, stress management, and exercise. Keto is a very powerful tool for weight loss, but it is only one piece of the puzzle. In order to successfully lose weight and keep it off, you need to start evaluating other areas of your life that may be holding you back from achieving your goals. In this book, I provide you with the proper tools and effective strategies to jump-start your healthier lifestyle and become the best version of yourself.

We will discuss why the standard recommendations for diet and weight loss are flawed, and you will learn exactly how to develop a well-formulated ketogenic protocol based on your individual needs and goals. You will learn how to effectively lose body fat while at the same time healing your body from the inside out and feeling amazing in the process. There are so many benefits to keto, but one of the main ones is that you can lose weight and become healthier while still enjoying delicious and satisfying food. The recipes provided in this book are easy to make, extremely flavorful, and easily adaptable to your preferences. One thing I hear often from my clients is, "I'm losing weight, I have so much energy, and the best part of it all is that I don't feel like I'm on a diet!"

In addition to more than 100 keto-friendly recipes, there are easy-to-follow meal plans that include lots of grab-and-go options, make-ahead tips, stream-lined shopping lists, and other helpful guidelines to make your transition to keto as easy as possible. You will find exercise routines and recommendations, goal-setting strategies, best practices for sleep and mind-set control, and tips for breaking bad habits. You'll gain a better understanding of how to manage everyday stressors, and you'll soon realize that making small changes along the way will lead to new, healthier habits and promote long-term results.

This challenge gives you the tools to jump-start your healthier lifestyle and provides tips and tricks that you can use during the 21 days and beyond. If at any time you feel overwhelmed or are having a difficult time with the transition, remember to take a step back and remind yourself why you started. Continue to embrace the positive changes you are making each day and realize that as long as you trust the process, you will succeed!

A NOTE FROM Amanda

I've had a lot of bad habits in my life. I smoked for years. I hung the toilet paper in the "under" position. I didn't wash peanut-buttery knives before putting them in the dishwasher.

But my worst habit was rewarding myself with food. And not just any food but the worst kinds of food. Finished a project? Pizza night! Working on chores? Soda! Laced my shoes correctly? Cake!

Meanwhile, I was poisoning myself and exacerbating every symptom of every internet-researched hypochondriac episode. It wasn't until I started testing out the ketogenic diet over a decade ago that I truly understood the words "you are what you eat."

My ketogenic journey started with a desire to lose weight, but it was my husband who first latched on to the idea when he began a bacon and butter diet, a diet I was sure would leave me a widow. He's the type to find something and then get really gung ho really quickly, so I tried to look up ways to dissuade him as fast as I could.

Instead, I found success story after success story and incredible research studies on the positive brain effects of the ketogenic diet.

I started the ketogenic diet thinking I could play it easy and simply toss the buns of my fast food burgers and eat almond flour brownies until my stomach exploded. But then I started feeling better on keto, and it made me want to improve my eating habits even more by focusing on consuming healthier fats.

That's when the ketogenic diet really started to improve my life. My chronic vertigo started to subside, as did other symptoms like anxiety. Soon I learned that if I was having a hard day, all I had to do was go hard on keto and I would feel better right away. My choices in food could cure my biggest daily challenges.

Since then, keto has simply become part of my life. I've enjoyed the weight-loss benefits of it, but I've benefited even more in my quality of life and state of mind.

My first book, *Keto Life*, was written as a guide for beginners, and my second, *The Wicked Good Ketogenic Diet Cookbook*, focused on the food. For this book, I was excited to team up with Rachel, with her taking the lead on setting an actionable plan for people new to the ketogenic diet. Rachel is a powerful force of knowledge on how to follow a ketogenic lifestyle consciously and with purpose.

As for my contribution to this gem of a book, I'm just here for the food, having contributed 25 recipes. All of the recipes are simple and easy to make, because something Rachel and I agree on is that to succeed with a ketogenic lifestyle, you have to keep it simple. The faster and easier you can make meal prep and cooking, the better.

That said, we all need a little spice in our lives to feel like we haven't dived into the deep end of plain chicken breasts, so you'll find recipes here that tickle your taste buds, too. Our goal in developing the recipes for this book came down to simplicity, whole ingredients, and familiarity. You'll find meal plans for real life, with plenty of options to make keto as easy as possible for you.

This book offers a genuine challenge, but it's only 21 days long. You can do anything for 21 days, and the best part is that you're taking a holistic approach to your health, which can only reap benefits. What we hope is that you'll achieve lasting results and that the changes to your diet and lifestyle will leave you with lasting good habits that continue to positively impact your life.

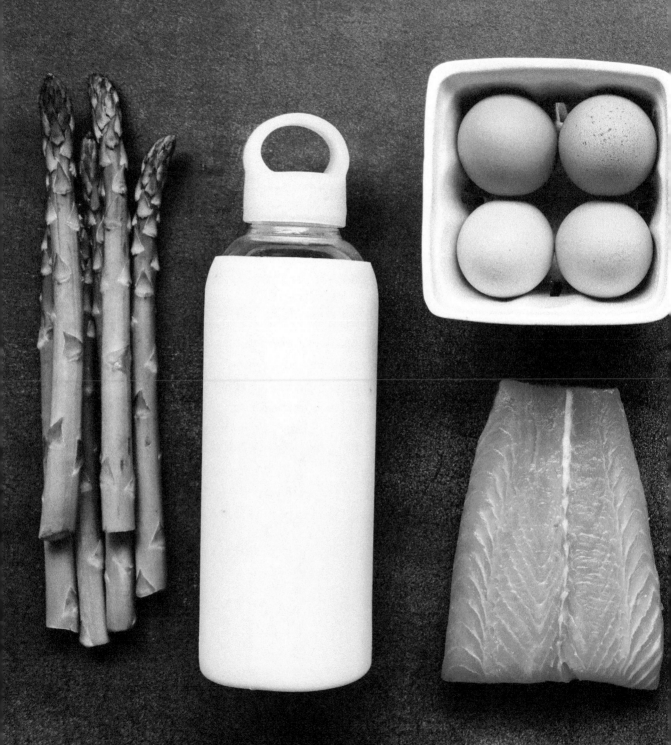

PART ONE

Your Keto Solution

STOP BLAMING YOURSELF for gaining weight or not being able to lose it. Throw everything you've learned about "healthy whole grains" and "heart-healthy" labels out the window. It's time to set the record straight and truly learn what a healthy, sustainable, and easy approach to weight loss entails.

In these next few chapters, you will learn why weight loss is not all about calories in, calories out; how a diet based on traditional dietary guidelines is flawed; and why eating fat does not have anything to do with "gaining fat." You will learn the proper way to fuel your body to become a "fat-burner" rather than a "sugar-burner," and you'll do all this while still enjoying foods that are filling, satisfying, delicious, and easy to prepare. After just 21 days, you'll have learned the foundations of a low-carbohydrate, ketogenic lifestyle and understand why it is not only maintainable, but also extremely enjoyable.

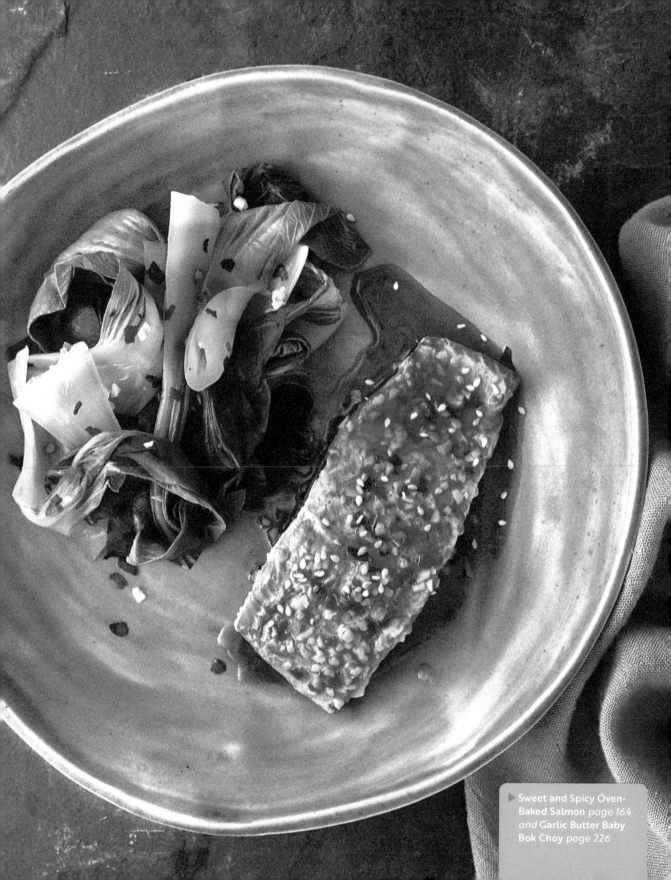

▶ Sweet and Spicy Oven-Baked Salmon *page 164 and* Garlic Butter Baby Bok Choy *page 226*

1

Ketogenic Diet and Weight Loss

I f you're looking for the answer to why two out of three Americans are currently overweight or obese, it's actually quite simple—we have all been fed misinformation for the past 50 years that has led to substantial increases in obesity, diet-related illnesses, and chronic diseases. We have been told to follow dietary guidelines that are inherently flawed and based on inaccurate research funded by industries that care more about their rising profit margins than the rise in chronic health problems.

As a result, our approach to achieving superior health and weight loss has been completely wrong for years. Although a diet focused around fruits, vegetables, and whole grains is far superior to one based on sugar and processed foods, many people still struggle to achieve lasting weight loss. This is where a low-carbohydrate, ketogenic lifestyle comes into play. By fueling our bodies in a way that allows access to body fat stores and prevents a constant rise and drop in blood sugar levels, we set ourselves up for a successful and lasting weight-loss journey.

▶ Problems with the Standard American Diet

The Standard American Diet, or "SAD" (pun intended), is based on nutritional guidelines (high carb, low fat) that put our bodies into a constant state of fat-storing rather than fat-burning. According to the United States Department of Agriculture (USDA) Dietary Guidelines, we are taught that carbohydrates are a necessary fuel source needed to maintain energy throughout the day. This could not be further from the truth. Carbohydrates, yes, even the "heart-healthy" complex ones such as whole grains, fruits, beans, potatoes, etc., are turned into sugar (or glucose) when consumed. This causes blood sugar levels to rise and signals the pancreas to release a hormone called insulin.

Insulin is needed to shuttle sugar (glucose) out of the blood and into cells because our bodies are only meant to handle a teaspoon (about 4 grams) of sugar in the bloodstream at one time. This is why insulin is known as the "fat storage hormone," because whenever insulin is around, it tells the body to store energy rather than use it. Once muscle and liver cells are filled to capacity with glucose (also referred to as "glycogen stores"), the remaining glucose is stored in fat cells.

The underlying problem with a high-carb diet is that the pancreas is over-worked when we continuously demand it to release insulin. Eventually, the pancreas stops releasing adequate amounts of insulin to keep up with the continual rise in blood sugar and the cells start to become resistant to the insulin that *is* produced. This causes a buildup of sugar in the bloodstream and eventually contributes to the development of type 2 diabetes, an epidemic plaguing our society today. Additionally, insulin resistance leads to weight gain, inflammation, and many chronic diseases and disorders. The bottom line is that we want to make sure our bodies are not on the path to insulin resistance and instead are working toward becoming more insulin sensitive, a process that occurs when we do not rely on carbohydrates as our main fuel source.

A CLOSER LOOK AT A "HEALTHY" WHOLE FOODS DIET

Have other diets claiming to be based on "healthy" whole foods failed you in the past? Well, you're not alone. We're taught that a healthy diet consists of oatmeal with fruit for breakfast, a turkey sandwich on whole-grain bread with a side of sliced apple for lunch, and a dinner consisting of lean chicken breast with a side of quinoa and veggies. Oh, and don't forget the low-fat yogurt, granola bars, and fruit for snacks throughout the day to "keep our metabolism going." Sounds pretty healthy, right? Let's take a quick look at the carbohydrate intake for this typical "healthy" day of eating:

- **Breakfast:** ½ cup oats prepared with 1 cup skim milk, ½ sliced banana, 1 cup fresh squeezed orange juice = 80g carbs

- **Snack:** 1 (4-ounce) container of low-fat strawberry yogurt with ¼ cup granola = 38g carbs

- **Lunch:** turkey sandwich on 2 whole-grain bread slices with 2 tablespoons low-fat mayo, 2 American cheese slices, and 1 medium apple = 71g carbs

- **Snack:** 1 granola bar = 26g carbs

- **Dinner:** 1 (4-ounce) chicken breast, ½ cup quinoa, ½ cup cooked peas and carrots = 30g carbs

- **Dessert:** 3 cups microwave popcorn, 1 large orange = 34g carbs

- **Total for Day:** 2,054 calories, 50g fat, 139g protein, 279g carbs

Consuming around 300 grams of carbohydrates, which is converted to 300 grams of sugar (or glucose) in the body, in one day and calling it a "healthy" diet is far from accurate (remember your pancreas can only handle 4 grams of sugar in the bloodstream at a time). Look at it this way: The same people who are promoting this diet are the ones slapping "heart-healthy" labels on processed junk like sugary cereal and chemically processed vegetable oils. I'm pretty sure eating a bowl of sugar for breakfast and cooking with highly processed, inflammatory oils is not what constitutes "heart-healthy." Take a step back and think about where these guidelines are coming from and who's actually benefiting from them. I'll give you a hint: It's not your waistline.

▶ Burn Fat, Not Sugar

If you look back at the history of our ancestors, you'll see that they consumed a diet that is the opposite of what we are told to consume today (low fat, high carb). Our bodies are inherently programmed to thrive on a high fat, low carb diet, and adopting a ketogenic lifestyle will allow your body to do just that.

A ketogenic diet consists of a low-carb, moderate-protein, high-fat approach to food and drink consumption. When you decrease your carbohydrate intake and subsequently increase your healthy fat intake, your body switches from a sugar-burning state to a fat-burning state, also known as ketosis.

Ketosis is the metabolic state of burning fat for fuel.

By decreasing your carb intake, you decrease the amount of glucose (sugar) entering your body and therefore decrease the need for a constant release of insulin (remember, insulin is the fat storage hormone). By doing this, you allow your body to tap into its fat stores and begin burning ketones and fatty acids for fuel rather than relying on glucose. To lose body fat, you need to burn it for energy. If you're constantly feeding your body carbs, you will have a hard time tapping into your body fat, making fat loss nearly impossible.

The scientific literature supporting a low-carbohydrate, ketogenic diet for weight loss is overwhelming. Several studies, including a review by Paoli et al. in the *European Journal of Clinical Nutrition*, have found that a ketogenic diet can lead to not only significant and sustainable weight loss, but also aid in the prevention and even possible reversal of several health-related diseases such as type 2 diabetes, metabolic syndrome, cancer, Alzheimer's, Parkinson's, epilepsy, fatty liver disease, and more.

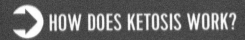
THE STANDARD AMERICAN DIET: HIGH CARB

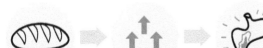

Eat a high carb diet

Blood sugar/ glucose levels rise

Pancreas releases insulin

Insulin shuttles glucose into cells

Burst of energy

Blood sugar crashes leading to cravings, hunger, lethargy

THE KETOGENIC DIET: LOW CARB

Eat a low carb, Keto diet

Blood sugar/ glucose levels fall

Fat cells release stored fatty acids

Fatty acids travel to liver, muscle, and other tissues

Liver converts fatty acids to ketones and muscle/tissues break fatty acids down for energy

Blood sugar and insulin levels low and stable. Fat is burned/ muscle is spared.

BUT ISN'T FAT BAD FOR YOU?

For years we have been demonizing fat as the enemy. We've been told that fat causes heart disease, weight gain, and a whole host of other health problems. But did you know, the claims surrounding "fat is bad" come from false and corrupted data produced by corporate and political influencers? Surprise, surprise.

A 2016 study published in the *Journal of the American Medical Association* revealed that one of the main culprits of this false information stemmed from the sugar industry funding studies in the 1960s and '70s that pointed the finger at fat while covering up the real evidence showing that sugar was actually the main cause of inflammation and many other health issues. It doesn't take an expert to figure this one out. The low-fat and fat-free trends that dominated the food industry in the 1980s stemmed from the fear of fat and the financial motive of the sugar industry. When you remove the fat from food, you take away the flavor. So, in order to get that flavor back, you have to add sugar. This flawed concept of "healthy" has led to the sugar industry profiting immensely while our society has gotten fatter and sicker.

Added to this was the replacement of real fats like butter and lard with factory-made vegetable and seed oils like margarine and canola oil that claim to be "heart-healthy" but in reality cause chronic inflammation and thus, more diseases! Based on statistics from the National Institute of Diabetes and Digestive and Kidney Diseases, it's no wonder two out of three Americans are overweight or obese, and more than 30.3 million have diabetes (compared to 1.6 million in 1958, before the "low-fat" craze began).

Interestingly, a recent 10-year study published in *The Lancet* looking at 135,000 adults from 18 countries found that those cutting back on fats like butter, cheese, and meat had shorter lives than those who enjoyed them. The study concluded "higher intake of fats, including saturated fats, is associated with lower risk of mortality."

The takeaway here is this: Fat is not the bad guy. Sugar, low-fat packaged foods, and highly processed grains are the enemy!

▶ Keto Principles

In order to successfully heal your body and lose weight following a ketogenic protocol, it's imperative that you understand the basic breakdown of macronutrients. Macronutrients (or "macros") are the basic components of food: carbohydrate, fat, and protein. On a well-formulated, whole foods–based ketogenic diet, like the one you'll find in this book, your macros should fall into this percentage range:

- 5 to 10 percent calories from carbohydrate (carbohydrate = 4 calories per gram)
- 15 to 30 percent calories from protein (protein = 4 calories per gram)
- 60 to 80 percent calories from fat (fat = 9 calories per gram)

LOW CARB

The most important macro to focus on when adopting a ketogenic lifestyle is carbohydrates. In order to get into ketosis and switch from being a "sugar-burner" to a "fat-burner," carbohydrate intake must be low. For the average person, this means keeping your carb intake to fewer than 30 total grams per day (20 grams for those who have severe metabolic damage or up to 50 grams, sometimes more, for those who are very active).

MODERATE PROTEIN

The amount of protein a person needs to consume on a well-formulated ketogenic diet is somewhat individualized based on factors such as body composition, intensity and frequency of exercise, specific health conditions, and more. In general, most people can remain in ketosis and achieve consistent results by consuming 0.8 grams of protein per pound of lean body mass. Lean body mass includes everything in your body that is not fat (muscle, water, bones, organs). This number is determined by subtracting your body fat from your total body weight. We will discuss how to determine your individual lean body mass in chapter 2.

HIGH FAT

The last piece of the puzzle is getting enough fat from healthy sources to make up for the reduction in the other two food groups. There is a lot of controversy surrounding the consumption of dietary fat when you're trying to lose weight on a keto diet. From my experience, if you are just beginning this journey and drastically reducing carb intake while also keeping your fat intake low, you will most likely feel terrible and give up after a week. This is because you're asking your body to switch from using a fuel that it has been using its whole life (sugar) to fuels that it barely knows how to use (fat and ketones). Increasing your intake of dietary fat will help ease the transition. Once your body gets used to burning fat and ketones for fuel, it will begin to tap into its own body fat stores and break them down for fuel instead of relying on dietary fat.

Don't make this harder than it has to be. Just reduce your carbohydrate intake and consume protein and fat to fill the gap. Consuming healthy fats will give you energy, keep you satiated, and help regulate your hormones as you adjust to this new lifestyle. As you progress, you'll notice that your body starts to feel fuller, faster, and you will naturally reduce the amount of food you eat as your body starts to tap into its existing fat stores and use them for energy.

▶ The Benefits

There are many benefits to following a high-quality, whole food–based ketogenic lifestyle and becoming keto-adapted. I like to say that weight and fat loss is just an added bonus on top of all the other benefits that lead to a higher quality of life.

Sustained weight loss and improved body composition: Not only has a ketogenic diet proven successful for substantial fat and weight loss in a relatively short period of time, but unlike other diets, a ketogenic protocol has also shown to be sustainable and enjoyable. Weight loss means nothing if you can't keep it off in the long term and that is why so many people have found success when adopting a ketogenic lifestyle.

Improved energy and mood: Because fat and ketones provide a readily available source of energy and keto helps stabilize blood sugar and insulin levels in your body, you won't experience the constant dips and spikes in these levels through-out the day. This leads to a higher yet stable energy level and enhanced mood all day long.

Improved cognitive function, mental clarity, focus, and memory: This is proba-bly the benefit I love the most! Being in a state of ketosis allows your brain to function at its optimal level while simultaneously protecting your brain for long-term health. The human brain is made up of nearly 60 percent fat, so it's no surprise that our brains actually prefer and thrive with adequate fat and ketones.

Improved insulin sensitivity and decreased inflammation: Switching from being a sugar-burner to being a fat and ketone–burner reduces both the reliance on high insulin production and the amount of reactive oxygen species (ROS) in your body that cause damage and inflammation—the primary driver of chronic disease.

Enhanced recovery and increased performance: Reduced inflammation, enhanced energy production and efficiency, muscle preservation, and cellular protection are just a few of the outcomes of being in a state of ketosis that result in improved recovery times between workouts and overall increases in exercise performance over the long term.

Disease prevention and treatment: The evidence continues to emerge as the ketogenic diet proves successful in reducing the severity of, and even reversing, common diseases like epilepsy, diabetes, heart disease, nonalcoholic fatty liver disease, Alzheimer's, Parkinson's, cancer, and others.

Stabilized hormones: When keto-adaptation occurs, many hormones in your body begin to heal and stabilize. This leads to various benefits including appetite control, enhanced fertility outcomes, fewer cravings, more energy, sustained weight loss, and much more.

Anti-aging and enhanced quality of life: The lowering of oxidative stress and inflammation paired with the balancing of blood sugar, insulin, and hormonal levels are just some of the key factors that demonstrate the anti-aging power of keto.

▶ The 21-Day Keto Challenge

The goal of this 21-day keto challenge is to kick-start your new keto lifestyle with a focus on weight and fat loss that is healthy and sustainable. The idea of following a specific diet protocol can be daunting, even overwhelming, for many people. This book will help by giving you a comprehensive plan that is simple yet effective and takes the guesswork out of meal planning while at the same time providing the education and fundamentals you need to be successful in the long term.

Whether you are new to keto, are looking to get back on track with keto, or have tried keto and didn't get the results you were hoping for, this challenge can help. Many people who start a ketogenic protocol fail to achieve their goals because they are bogged down by misinformation. The accurate information and detailed plan in this book will simplify keto and provide what you need to know in a way that is easy to understand, follow, and adapt to your specific needs.

Additionally, as a bonus feature to this book, you will receive a discount code to join the online 21-Day Keto Challenge that provides a day-to-day accountability system, virtual community setting with like-minded participants, and access to work directly with me for further support, guidance, motivation, and trouble-shooting advice. Many of my clients came to me with tales of previously failing to reach their goals because a support and accountability system was not there. My hope is that you will use this book as your starting guide and pair it with the online program to provide the missing pieces of daily accountability, community support, and professional guidance. You can visit my website at www.killinitketo.com to learn more about this program and browse the testimonials from former clients who provided their stories of success and lasting results. The special discount for book owners can be found at www.killinitketo.com/book-owner.

More than just a meal plan, the keto challenge offers a holistic approach to health and weight loss, including five fundamental pillars:

1. Nutrition

2. Exercise

3. Sleep

4. Stress management

5. Mind-set

Achieving lasting weight loss and, more importantly, optimized health is not just about what you eat or how much you exercise. Your body is a very smart machine, and if you're not giving it the proper care and nourishment it needs, you'll continue to fall short of achieving your health goals. During this 21-day keto challenge you will actively focus on all aspects of physical, mental, and emotional well-being by learning strategies that can easily be implemented into your every-day life. We'll dive into each one in more detail in the chapters to come.

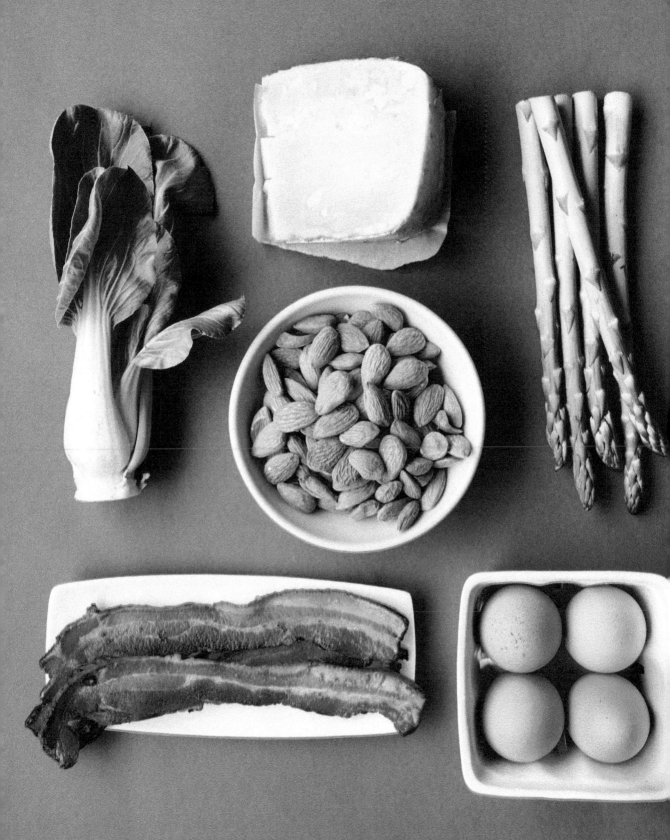

2

Keto Nutrition

There's a saying out there that weight loss is 80 percent nutrition and 20 percent exercise. I disagree. I believe that *sustained* and *healthy* weight loss cannot be divided into a set ratio because there are so many more pieces to the puzzle. Mind-set, stress, hormonal balance, sleep, physical activity, food quality, food quantity, social surroundings, and other lifestyle factors all play a role in your ability to lose weight, and more importantly, keep that weight off.

However, if I were to choose the piece of the puzzle that plays the largest role, it would be what you put in your mouth on a daily basis. In this chapter, we will discuss the first pillar of your keto challenge: nutrition. You'll learn exactly what types and ratios of foods to consume, steps to ensure an easy transition into keto-adaptation, and an overall understanding of how to successfully implement keto for weight loss.

▶ All About Ratios

When starting keto, many people make the mistake of thinking they can consume copious amounts of calories and fat. Then they question why they are not seeing the scale move or feel their pants getting looser. It's important to realize that although calories are not the be-all and end-all, if you're consuming more energy than your body needs and uses, it must be stored somewhere.

Keto helps you lose weight and keep it off because it helps stabilize your blood sugar and insulin levels so you're not constantly searching for food all day. Keto allows you to feel completely satiated while dulling cravings, it increases your overall energy and mood so you naturally become more active, and it ultimately heals your body from the inside out by providing more efficient and effective fuel sources—fat and ketones. So while you'll still want to keep track of calories, when transitioning to a keto diet you'll be focusing a lot more on the ratio of fat, protein, and carbs that make up your meals. All of the recipes and meal plans in this book provide a balanced ratio of keto macros to help you easily adjust to this lifestyle.

MACRONUTRIENT RATIOS FOR WEIGHT LOSS

"Carbs are a limit, protein is a goal, and fat is a lever"—this is a common saying that circulates around our keto community. In general, this is how you will structure your macros throughout the day.

How Many Carbs?

5 to 10 percent calories from carbohydrate (carbohydrate = 4 calories per gram)
Aiming for **30 grams total carbs or less per day** is a good place to start and generally gets people into ketosis and helps them stay there. Sometimes 20 grams or less is necessary for those who have severe metabolic damage, and up to 50 grams, sometimes more, for those who are very active. See Counting Carbs on page 20 for more detail on how to track carb intake.

How Much Protein?

15 to 30 percent calories from protein (protein = 4 calories per gram)

Determining protein intake can take a little bit more work because it is highly individualized.

Ideal approach: In general, most people can remain in ketosis and achieve consistent results by consuming **0.8 grams of protein per pound of lean body mass** (see Body Composition Analysis on page 18 for how to determine your lean body mass). Those who are more active may benefit from bumping up to 1.0 or 1.2 grams of protein per pound of lean body mass.

Quick and dirty approach: If you don't know your lean body mass number or don't feel like doing the math, **dividing your body weight (in pounds) in half** is usually a good place to start for determining moderate protein intake. For example, if you weigh 230 pounds, divide 230 by 2 to get 115. Your protein goal would be around 115 grams total per day. Note: if you are sedentary and have a history of metabolic damage, you may need to lower this number by 15 to 20 grams to achieve nutritional ketosis.

Your daily protein intake will most likely need to be adjusted as you progress through this lifestyle change and discover the amount of protein you can consume while staying in ketosis, feeling good, and getting results.

How Much Fat?

60 to 80 percent calories from fat (fat = 9 calories per gram)

If you keep your carbs low and hit your protein goal, the last piece to work out is fat intake. The specific amount of fat you consume will be based on the remaining calories left in your day (once you've subtracted the carbs and protein).

Ideally, if you hit your carb and protein intake and eat fat to true satiety, you'll begin to heal your body and lose the unnecessary and unwanted body fat. Sounds simple, right? Well, it may be . . . for those people who are in tune with their satiety levels, are not prone to overeating, and have natural portion control. But, as most of us reading this book know, it's not that simple, especially when we've gone through years of yo-yo dieting, deprivation, and eating foods that are completely devoid of the nutrients needed to balance our hormone levels.

Although there is really no 100 percent accurate way to determine how many calories a particular person burns in one day, there are formulas and online

➡ BODY COMPOSITION ANALYSIS

How do you measure body fat percentage and determine lean body mass?

There are several ways to measure body fat, but the most accurate is a DEXA scan. Other methods include whole body plethysmography (Bod Pod), underwater/hydrostatic weighing, bioelectrical impedance analysis (BIA or the popular InBody scanner), skinfold calipers, body tape measurements, or visual estimation guides (photos). It's important to note that these methods differ in their accuracy and you should focus on consistency when using them to track progress. Many gyms, health centers, and even some doctors' offices offer body composition analyses, and it's as simple as an internet search for those offered in your area and choosing the one that fits your budget.

For practical and cost-effective purposes, measuring at home can still offer pretty good results. Simply purchase a tape measure and do an internet search for the "US Navy Body Fat Calculator" (see Resources, page 264). Follow the directions, entering your information and measurements when prompted.

You can also do an internet search for "body fat visual estimation guides" to use as a comparative method to your own body composition (it's best to overestimate rather than underestimate when using this method).

Once you determine your body fat percentage, you can easily figure out your lean body mass. Simply multiply the decimal equivalent of your body fat percentage by your body weight in pounds. For example, if your body fat is 35 percent and you weigh 180 pounds, multiply 0.35 by 180 pounds = 63 pounds. This is your fat mass or the amount of fat

calculators that can be used to estimate caloric needs based on gender, age, height, weight, body fat percentage, and daily activity level.

There are several online nutrition calculators out there, with some being more accurate than others. For an in-depth keto calculator, check out ankerl.com, and for a simpler version, visit mariamindbodyhealth.com and search "keto calculator." Just input your numbers and use the outcome as a guide to determine an appropriate starting point for your individual caloric intake and keto macros.

Alternatively, and my recommendation when first starting this challenge, download a food tracking application such as Senza, which is completely free

(63 pounds) you have on your body. Now, to determine your lean body mass, subtract your fat mass from your total body weight (180 − 63 = 117 pounds). This means you have 117 pounds of lean body mass. So, to determine your ideal protein intake based on 0.8 grams of protein per pound of lean body mass, you would multiply 117 x 0.8 = 94 grams of protein per day or

376 calories of protein per day (1 gram of protein is equivalent to 4 calories, 94 x 4 = 376 calories). As you can see, if you had just divided the weight (180 pounds) by 2, you would have calculated a slightly less accurate 90 grams of protein per day. Go ahead and fill in your numbers below to make this easier.

WEIGHT: _____ BODY FAT PERCENTAGE: _____

WEIGHT _____ X BODY FAT DECIMAL AMOUNT _____ = _____ FAT MASS

WEIGHT _____ – FAT MASS _____ = _____ LEAN BODY MASS

LEAN BODY MASS _____ X 0.8 GRAMS OF PROTEIN PER POUND OF LEAN BODY MASS

= _____ GRAMS OF PROTEIN PER DAY

Confused? No worries, just take that body fat percentage number and head over to an online keto calculator (see page 265 for more info on this) or the Senza application (see page 265) to determine a guide for figuring out your starting macros for the challenge.

to use and specific to the ketogenic lifestyle (this is the application I use with my clients and can be found by doing a quick search in your phone's app store). You can input your information into the app's calculator to find an appropriate starting point for your calorie and macronutrient goals.

A few notes on these nutrition calculators:

1. Most of these calculators suggest tracking net carbs instead of total carbs. See the Counting Carbs sidebar (page 20) for why I believe tracking total carbs is more accurate, especially when you're starting out.

2. Some of the online keto calculators implement an extreme reduction in caloric intake when setting weight loss as a goal. I recommend focusing on changing the composition of your macros first (lower carbs, moderate protein, increased fat) and then reduce your calories as you start to become naturally satiated and full. If you immediately reduce your calories while at the same time trying to change the metabolic fuel that your body is accustomed to using (sugar) over to fat, problems can arise such as feeling horrible and experiencing extreme symptoms of "keto flu" (page 40). We want this weight loss to be sustainable, and in order for that to happen, you have to allow your body some time to adjust.

3. Make sure to double-check and align your daily carb and protein intake with the suggestions outlined previously.

→ COUNTING CARBS

I believe that when first starting a ketogenic protocol, it's important to focus on total carbs rather than net carbs (net carbs = total carbs − fiber). Some people would disagree, but I have found that it's much easier and more reliable, especially in the beginning, to concentrate on the total grams of carbohydrate intake. This removes the guesswork and eliminates falling into the trap of over-consuming hidden carbs or food products that claim to have a "low net carb" count but in reality can spike blood sugar and insulin, holding you back from your health and weight-loss goals. The one exception to this rule pertains to green leafy vegetables and avocados. Because they are nutrient-dense and very high in fiber, counting net carbs for these (remember,

net carbs = total carbs − fiber) is okay as long as you don't go too crazy with them.

All of the recipes and meal plans in this book have a low total carb count, making it easy to cook and enjoy meals without worrying about exceeding your total daily carbohydrate intake. However, when you're eating out at restaurants or prepping other meals, it's important to be mindful of the amount of carbs in your food. Using a food tracking app can be helpful when planning meals and figuring out the amount of carbs in different food and drink items. Again, the app Senza is very helpful. It's free, specific to the ketogenic lifestyle, user-friendly, and has several features to help you stay on track. It also offers the option to track total or net carbs, which is a huge plus in my book.

MICRONUTRIENTS

In addition to balancing macronutrients, it's important to also remember that micronutrients (vitamins and minerals) play a large role in maintaining vital bodily functions. Many people believe that most micronutrients come from fruits and vegetables. However, the reality is that the most nutrient-dense foods are animal proteins like beef and fish (and the *most* nutrients are found in their organs . . . beef liver anyone?).

If you're not a fan of organ meat, make sure to focus on consuming high-quality sources of whole foods like pasture-raised, grass-finished meats, dairy, and bone broth; wild-caught, sustainably sourced seafood; and organic vegetables when possible.

We'll get into the importance of specific minerals (electrolytes) at the end of this chapter, so stay tuned.

PORTION CONTROL

Being aware of portion sizes for common foods can be helpful and eye-opening. Here are some portion size guidelines to keep in mind:

FIST	PALM	HANDFUL	THUMB	THUMB TIP
1 cup	3–4 ounces	1 ounce	1 ounce or 1–2 tablespoons	1–2 teaspoons
Raw, non-starchy vegetables	Meat Fish Poultry	Nuts Seeds Olives	Cheese Nut Butter	Oils Butter

▶ What to Eat

Now that you've determined your macros, it's time to discuss the different types of foods you'll be enjoying during this challenge and throughout your keto journey. The keto food guide pyramid below inverts the typical USDA pyramid with the majority of calories coming from healthy fat and protein.

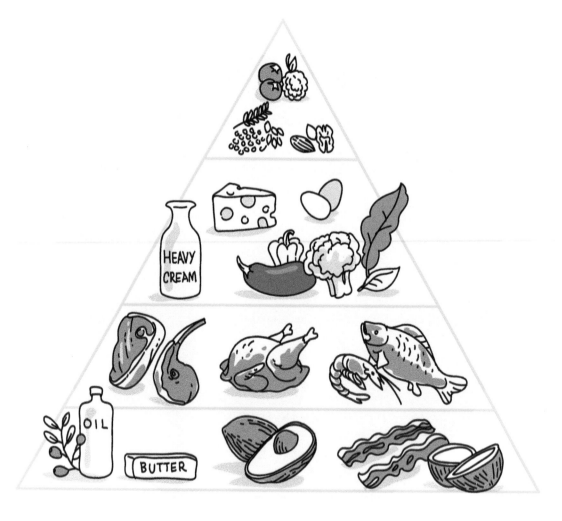

HEALTHY FATS

Fats will make up the majority of your daily food intake so it's important to choose the right ones. Fats are divided into four categories: saturated, mono-unsaturated, polyunsaturated, and trans fats. You'll want to consume saturated and monounsaturated fats often, polyunsaturated fats sparingly, and avoid trans fats as much as possible.

Saturated fats such as coconut oil, MCT oil, ghee, butter, tallow, and lard and other animal fats such as bacon, beef, and duck are the most stable fats, meaning they are less likely to oxidize or go rancid and cause increased inflammation in your body. Choose 100 percent grass-fed and organic when possible.

Monounsaturated fats like avocados, olives, nuts, seeds, avocado oil, and olive oil are moderately stable and best consumed in their whole food state or minimally processed. When buying these oils, look for ones in dark bottles and labeled "cold-pressed," "expeller-pressed," or "centrifuge-extracted."

Polyunsaturated fats such as canola, soybean, safflower, corn, grapeseed, and sunflower oil should be avoided because they are highly processed and prone to oxidation, leading to increased inflammation in the body. Focusing on whole food sources of omega-3 polyunsaturated fats, like salmon, sardines, walnuts, hemp seeds, and chia seeds, is a much safer and healthier option.

Trans fats like hydrogenated or partially hydrogenated oils, margarine, and vegetable shortening should be avoided at all costs. Trans fats are extremely inflammatory and have been linked to several health issues.

PROTEIN

When choosing protein sources, it is always best to find options that contain the least number of added hormones, antibiotics, and other harmful toxins. When possible, choose 100 percent grass-fed and -finished, pasture-raised, organic meat and dairy, and wild-caught seafood.

Your main sources of protein will include red meat, poultry, seafood, eggs, and dairy; smaller amounts from nuts, seeds, and vegetables; and limited fruits. Bone broth, collagen, and gelatin are also great sources of protein that are packed with beneficial nutrients.

NON-STARCHY VEGETABLES, LOW-SUGAR FRUITS, AND OTHER CARBOHYDRATES

The majority of your carbohydrate intake will come from non-starchy veggies, low-sugar fruits, nuts and seeds, and the small amounts present in dairy and other sources like dressings and sauces, condiments, beverages, and herbs and spices.

Non-starchy veggies include those that mostly grow above ground, like leafy greens, cabbage, broccoli, cauliflower, and others. Low-sugar fruits to enjoy include avocados, cucumbers, olives, eggplant, and smaller amounts of tomatoes and berries. Also, enjoy fermented foods like sauerkraut, kimchi, pickles, kefir, and small amounts of high-quality kombucha.

The grams of carbohydrates add up quickly throughout the day, so it helps to focus on sticking with whole food sources and avoiding packaged or processed foods. Of course, you'll have some keto-friendly pantry staples and other miscellaneous foods and drinks to enjoy, but the majority of your diet should contain items that are *as close to nature as possible*.

▶ Complete Keto Foods List

The following is a complete list of foods, beverages, and other low-carb options to enjoy. Please see the Keto-Specific Staples on page 28 for a detailed description, tips for best options when purchasing, and recommended brands for many of the ingredients listed.

REFRIGERATOR AND FREEZER

Meat

- Beef
- Chicken
- Cured meats—bacon, pancetta, pepperoni, prosciutto, etc.
- Duck
- Lamb
- Organ meats
- Pork
- Sausage
- Turkey

Eggs

- Chicken
- Duck
- Goose
- Quail

Fish/Seafood

- Anchovies
- Catfish
- Clams
- Cod
- Crab
- Flounder
- Haddock
- Halibut
- Lobster
- Mackerel
- Mahi mahi
- Oysters
- Salmon
- Sardines
- Scallops
- Shrimp
- Squid
- Swordfish
- Tuna

Dairy

- Butter
- Cheese
- Cottage cheese (in moderation)
- Cream cheese
- Heavy cream
- Kefir (in moderation)
- Labneh (Greek-style cheese)
- Mascarpone cheese
- Plain Greek yogurt (in moderation)
- Ricotta cheese (in moderation)
- Sour cream

Milk Substitutes

- Almond milk
- Cashew milk
- Coconut milk
- Hemp milk
- Macadamia nut milk

Vegetables

- Artichokes
- Arugula
- Asparagus
- Bok choy
- Broccoli
- Broccoli rabe
- Brussels sprouts (in moderation)
- Cabbage
- Carrots (in moderation)
- Cauliflower (whole and riced)
- Celery
- Collard greens
- Endive
- Fresh herbs (basil, cilantro, parsley, etc.)
- Garlic
- Green beans
- Kale
- Kimchi
- Lettuce (romaine, Boston, red leaf, radicchio)
- Mushrooms
- Onions (scallions, red, white, yellow) (in moderation)
- Peppers (bell, chile, jalapeño) (in moderation)
- Pickles
- Pumpkin (in moderation)
- Radishes
- Sauerkraut
- Spaghetti squash (in moderation)
- Spinach
- Swiss chard
- Zucchini (whole and noodles)
- Watercress

Fruit

- Avocado
- Berries (limited quantities)
- Coconut (unsweetened)
- Cucumber
- Eggplant
- Lemons
- Limes
- Olives
- Tomatoes (in moderation)

Nuts and Seeds, Nut/Seed Butters, and Flours

- Almond butter (unsweetened)
- Almond flour
- Almonds
- Brazil nuts
- Chia seeds
- Coconut flour
- Flaxseed
- Hazelnuts
- Hemp seeds
- Macadamia nuts
- Peanut butter (made from just peanuts and salt)
- Peanuts
- Pecans
- Pili nuts (best keto nut!)
- Pine nuts
- Pumpkin seeds
- Sesame seeds
- Sunflower seeds
- Walnuts

Beverages

- Bone broth
- Iced coffee
- Iced tea (unsweetened)
- Water (still and sparkling)
- Zevia (stevia-sweetened soda)

Condiments, Sauces, and Flavorings

- Barbecue sauce (sugar-free)
- Blue cheese dressing
- Caesar dressing
- Coconut aminos
- Fish sauce
- Harissa paste
- Horseradish
- Ketchup (sugar-free)
- Liquid aminos
- Mayonnaise (made with healthy oil like avocado or olive)
- Mustard (Dijon, spicy, yellow)
- Pesto
- Ranch dressing

PANTRY

Fats and Oils

- Avocado oil
- Bacon fat
- Beef tallow
- Cacao butter
- Chicken fat (schmaltz)
- Coconut butter/manna
- Coconut oil
- Duck fat
- Ghee
- Goose fat
- Lard
- Macadamia nut oil
- MCT oil/powder
- Olive oil (extra-virgin)
- Sesame oil (in moderation)

Vinegars and Other Flavorings

- Apple cider vinegar
- Balsamic vinegar (limited amounts)
- Coconut vinegar
- Hot sauce
- Maple extract (sugar-free)
- Nutritional yeast
- Red wine vinegar
- Tomato paste (in a tube)
- Tomato sauce (lowest sugar option)
- Vanilla extract, pure
- Water/electrolyte enhancers

Jarred, Canned, and Others

- Artichoke hearts (in moderation)
- Beef jerky or sticks (sugar-free)
- Boxed broth/stock
- Cheese crisps
- Coconut cream, unsweetened
- Coconut milk, unsweetened
- Green chiles
- Pickled jalapeños
- Pork rinds
- Olives, jarred
- Seafood, canned (anchovies, mackerel, salmon, sardines, tuna)
- Shirataki noodles and rice
- Tomatoes, crushed/diced and sauce (lowest sugar option, choose jarred over canned since the acid in tomatoes can draw potentially harmful chemicals from the can lining)

Herbs and Spices

For all herbs and spices, fresh and dried are acceptable. Choose organic, buy in bulk, and make "In a Hurry" Spice Blends (page 236).

- Allspice
- Basil
- Bay leaves
- Caraway
- Cardamom
- Celery seed
- Chili powder
- Chives
- Cilantro
- Cinnamon
- Cloves
- Coriander
- Cumin
- Curry
- Dill
- Garlic
- Ginger
- Marjoram
- Nutmeg
- Oregano
- Paprika
- Parsley
- Pepper, black
- Pepper, cayenne
- Pepper, red flakes
- Rosemary
- Sage
- Sea salt (Himalayan, Celtic)
- Tarragon
- Thyme
- Turmeric

Baking Products and Others

- Baking powder (aluminum-free)
- Baking soda
- Cacao butter, unsweetened
- Cacao/cocoa powder, unsweetened
- Cacao nibs, unsweetened
- Chocolate chips (sugar-free)
- Chocolate or cacao wafers, 100 percent dark
- Coconut chips/flakes, unsweetened
- Collagen powder
- Cream of tartar
- Gelatin, grass-fed, unflavored
- Guar gum
- MCT oil/powder
- Xanthan gum

Natural Sweeteners

- Erythritol
- Monk fruit
- Stevia

▶ Keto-Specific Staples

Here you'll find descriptions and recommended brands for several keto staples as well as suggestions for how to choose the best ones. You can also visit the Keto Alternatives page on my website (www.killinitketo.com/keto-alternatives) to learn more about these specialty keto products and find various discounts and brands that I recommend.

Meat and eggs: Choose 100 percent grass-fed and -finished, organic, free-range, hormone- and antibiotic-free, and/or pasture-raised when possible. Watch out for added sugars and fillers in bacon, sausage, and other cured meats. Check labels and choose meats with the least amount of sugar and without strange chemicals that you don't recognize.

Fish and seafood: Choose wild-caught and sustainably sourced seafood when possible. Buying frozen wild-caught seafood may be more cost effective and usually better quality unless you are getting it right from the fishing boat. Check out www.seafoodwatch.org to find the healthiest and most eco-friendly options.

Dairy: Choose full-fat dairy products, preferably 100 percent grass-fed and -finished, raw, and pasture-raised. Avoid buying packaged, shredded cheese because it has added starch (more carbs) to keep it from sticking together. Buy blocks of cheese and shred it yourself. Consume cottage cheese, ricotta, and plain yogurt in moderation because they are higher in carbs. Avoid processed cheeses like American or Velveeta. I use salted butter for just about everything. I like the Kerrygold Salted Butter (from grass-fed cows) that I buy in bulk at Costco. Feel free to use unsalted butter if you prefer, but note that in some recipes, you may need to add additional salt.

Vegetables: The rule of thumb is if it grows above ground, it's usually okay. The vegetables labeled "in moderation" should be consumed in smaller quantities because they have more carbs.

Cauliflower rice is a staple in my ketogenic kitchen. You can find frozen cauliflower rice in pretty much every grocery store nowadays. I keep at least three bags in my freezer at all times. Zucchini noodles (zoodles) are another staple. I use a spiralizer to make a big batch of zoodles at the beginning of the week and store them wrapped in a paper towel in the refrigerator for a quick side dish. Moderate your intake of Brussels sprouts, carrots, onions, peppers, pumpkin, and squash because they are higher in carbs.

Fruits: Most fruits should be avoided, especially during the first few weeks. One of the exceptions to this rule is my personal favorite food—avocados. Although avocados have slightly higher carbs, they are packed with healthy fats, fiber, and nutrients, making them a keto superfood. Limit berries and moderate your intake of tomatoes as the carbs add up quickly.

Nuts and seeds, nut/seed butters, and flours: I store all of my nuts and seeds, and anything made from them, in the refrigerator or freezer to prevent them from going rancid. Nuts and seeds are a great snack but they are very calorically dense and do have some carbs. A rule I like to stick to is limiting them to one or two servings per day (including nut/seed butters and flours). Pili nuts are my favorite and the most keto-friendly nut out there with only 1 gram of total carbs per ¼ cup (visit my website for more info on where to purchase them). Avoid pistachios and cashews because they are higher in carbs. Almond and coconut flour are staples in my keto kitchen and great for baking and cooking.

Beverages: Stock your refrigerator with sparkling waters or stevia-sweetened sodas like Zevia to replace any soda, juice, or other high-carb, sugary drinks. Brew a large batch of unsweetened tea for the week and add a dash sweetener if desired. Avoid milk and use heavy cream or unsweetened nut milks as creamers for your coffee.

Condiments, sauces, and flavorings: Always choose the lowest carb option made with a healthy fat source. Avoid anything made with inflammatory oils such as vegetable, canola, safflower, or sunflower oil. Choose salad dressings and mayonnaise made with avocado oil or make your own MCT oil–based dressing from scratch (see Fat-Burning Dressing on page 238). I like the Primal Kitchen and AlternaSweets brands of ketchup and barbecue sauce made with stevia, and I recommend using coconut aminos and liquid aminos as a healthier alternative to soy sauce. Use water/electrolyte powder enhancers such as Ultima Replenisher, Everly Hydration, or Stur to add flavor to your water while getting some extra electrolytes in.

Fats and oils: Choose 100 percent grass-fed, free-range, cold-pressed, pasture-raised where applicable. Stick with the fats and oils listed on page 27. Avoid any others, as they are probably highly inflammatory. As you become keto-adapted, these fats will be your body's primary fuel source, so it's important to incorporate them into your diet. MCT, or "medium-chain triglyceride" oil or powder, is a staple keto fat source because it is converted to ketones much faster than other saturated fats and therefore is a great tool for promoting keto-adaptation. MCTs can be used in a variety of recipes both savory and sweet or simply added to your morning coffee for an extra boost.

Jarred, canned, and others: Keeping your pantry stocked with keto-friendly options is very important for helping you stay on track. Sustainable and wild-caught canned seafood (Wild Planet brand, for example), sugar-free beef jerky or sticks, cheese crisps, and pork rinds (Bacon's Heir and EPIC are my favorite brands) are perfect for on-the-go options or snacks when you need them. Shirataki noodles and rice (Miracle Noodles brand is what I use) are other keto kitchen staples that are amazing alternatives to high-carb pasta and rice. They absorb the flavor of any dish and are extremely filling due to the high water and fiber content.

Baking products: There is a variety of different keto baking products on page 28 that may seem foreign at first but will become staples in your pantry to replace traditional flour, sugar, chocolate, cornstarch, and other ingredients. I use collagen and MCT powder in a lot of my recipes and recommend the Perfect Keto brand because they offer unflavored and flavored versions made with high-quality ingredients (visit the Keto Alternatives page on my website, www.killinitketo.com, for more information). Gelatin, guar gum, and xanthan gum can be used as thickeners in sauces, soups, and other recipes. Finding unsweetened, high-quality cacao butter or chocolate and using a natural sweetener (see below) is the best way to satisfy a sweet tooth without added sugar. Always choose aluminum-free baking powder.

Sweeteners: When purchasing sweeteners, make sure to read the ingredient labels thoroughly. Many companies add bulking ingredients such as dextrose and maltodextrin or use sugar alcohols like maltitol and sorbitol, all of which can actually raise your blood sugar levels and cause digestive issues—not good! I'd also avoid artificial sweeteners like aspartame, acesulfame potassium (Equal), sucralose (Splenda), and saccharin (Sweet'N Low) as much as possible. Pure monk fruit and stevia are my go-to sweeteners, but it's best to test for yourself and see which you prefer. Below are descriptions of some common keto-friendly sweeteners.

Monk fruit and stevia: These natural sweeteners are available in both liquid and powder form and are about 300 times sweeter than table sugar. Most of the powder forms on the market contain the bulking agents mentioned previously, so it's best to choose the liquid form or find a company that offers a pure extract powder. My favorite is the 80 percent monk fruit (also known as *luo han guo*) extract powder from Z Natural Foods. It is very concentrated, so a tiny dash goes a long way. I also use the liquid form of stevia or the pure stevia extract powder from Steviva.

Erythritol: This sugar alcohol is about 70 percent as sweet as table sugar. It doesn't affect blood sugar levels and is almost completely absorbed before it reaches the colon. This means that it doesn't cause as much digestive discomfort as some of the other sugar alcohols out there (like maltitol or sorbitol). Erythritol tends to have a slight cooling sensation in the mouth, so it may take some getting used to. Also, it's mostly sold in a granulated form that doesn't dissolve very well in foods, so it's best to grind it into a powder using a coffee or spice grinder before use. It's a common ingredient in keto cakes, cookies, and other treats because it pretty much measures cup-for-cup like sugar whereas monk fruit and stevia are used in much smaller quantities. I use the Wholesome brand of erythritol or blended versions (see below).

Blended sweeteners: Some brands combine two or more sweeteners to help balance flavors. Another usual ingredient in blended sweeteners is oligosaccharides, or "inulin," which is a sweet, non-digestible, prebiotic fiber found in starchy root vegetables that generally does not affect blood sugar levels. Some of the current popular brands of blended sweeteners include Steviva, Swerve, and Lakanto.

▶ A Day of Keto Meals

There are several different options (and opinions) when it comes to structuring your daily meals. The bottom line is that there is no one-size-fits-all approach for this and it really comes down to your individual schedule, eating habits, and ultimately what allows you to feel most satisfied while maintaining a balanced keto macro intake.

From my personal experience and work with clients, I have learned that the most effective approach to this type of weight-loss program is to try to eliminate as many stressors as possible in the beginning while easing into a "typical" keto eating pattern as the weeks progress. So if you're used to eating three meals and

 EATING WINDOWS AND THE CHEWING PHENOMENON

There are many potential health benefits to adopting a daily intermittent fasting protocol (see the sidebar What Is Intermittent Fasting? on page 35), but there's another possible implication of this practice for weight loss. Some people argue that if you don't chew your food (drinking a fatty coffee instead, for example), you will not activate the feeling of fullness or satiety in your brain and this could lead to overeating.

However, from personal experience and from what I've gathered from other clients and coaches, once you chew that first bite of food, it can actually trigger you to want to continue chewing and therefore lead to more snacking and more food intake. So, if your goal is to lose weight and do so without feeling

hungry or reaching for snacks all day long, you could benefit from the following:

1. Adopting a ketogenic diet protocol.

2. Pushing your first meal (or at least the first meal that involves chewing) until later in the day.

3. Consuming coffee or tea with some added fat for breakfast (not a whole stick of butter but rather a tablespoon or two of MCT oil or powder, butter, ghee, coconut oil, or whatever healthy fat you prefer) and avoid chewing gum or mints. I like to also add a few tablespoons of collagen powder to my coffee or tea for its tremendous health benefits for skin, hair, nails, improved gut health, and much more.

two snacks each day, go into the first week with the same schedule, just making sure those meals and snacks are keto-approved. If you're used to skipping breakfast and eating later in the day, then do that.

Once you're past the first week and getting the hang of consuming fewer carbohydrates, adequate protein, and more healthy fats, you will most likely start to feel more satiated and notice that you can go for longer periods of time without eating or snacking while still maintaining high energy, mood, and focus levels.

Here's an example of a typical weekly progression that seems to work well for many people. (Note: Each option includes hitting your total macro and caloric intake as set from the guidelines, and snacks are on an "if needed" basis.)

Week 1: Eat 3 meals + 2 or 3 snacks, or skip breakfast and eat 2 meals + 2 or 3 snacks.

Week 2: Eat 2 meals + 1 or 2 snacks. Skip breakfast and consume just coffee or tea with a small amount of fat and eat lunch around noon or 1 p.m. If you're a night eater or dessert person, save 1 snack for after dinner, but try not to eat too close to bedtime.

Week 3: Eat 2 meals + 1 snack. Skip breakfast, consume just coffee or tea with some added healthy fat, and eat lunch around 2 p.m. If you're a night eater or dessert person, save your snack for after dinner, but try not to eat too close to bedtime.

Making it a lifestyle: Figure out the meal timing that fits your personal schedule, keeps you feeling satisfied throughout the day, and allows you to enjoy your meals without triggering more stressors.

As we discussed earlier, the more snacking you do during the day, the more you trigger an insulin response (remember, insulin is the fat storage hormone). This is why intermittent fasting is so effective for weight loss and restoring insulin sensitivity; it prevents the constant elevation of insulin levels, leading to more healing and a greater ability to tap into those fat stores for energy. Ideally, you'd want to transition to two or three keto-based meals (or for some people even one large meal) with minimal snacking. But don't feel like you need to start with this as it can be another added stressor and cause a drop in long-term adherence.

WHAT IS INTERMITTENT FASTING?

When people hear the word "fasting," they often associate it with deprivation, restriction, and muscle wasting. However, those outcomes are definitely not the case with Intermittent Fasting (or IF as it's commonly called). IF is an eating pattern where you alternate between periods of fasting and feeding. There are several different protocols for IF, but the general idea is that you set a time window for eating, eat only within that window, and fast the remainder of the time. For example, eating only from noon to 8 p.m. would be considered the 16/8 method (16 hours fasting/8 hours feeding) or eating nothing from dinner one night until dinner the next night would be considered the Alternate Day Fasting method (24-hour fast). My favorite is a Fat Fasting protocol where you consume a small amount of healthy fats during your fasting window, which seems to increase adherence for many people while still gaining several of the fasting benefits (so long as you're not consuming an entire stick of butter in your morning coffee). Aim for a few tablespoons of healthy fats.

Some benefits of intermittent fasting:

- Stimulates brain function and enhances mental clarity
- Improves blood glucose control and insulin sensitivity
- Boosts ketone production
- Saves time with meal planning and preparation
- Accelerates weight loss and fat-burning
- Reduces inflammation and potentially slows aging and disease processes

Note: If you are someone who does better eating earlier in the day and having your last meal around 5 or 6 p.m., that is totally fine and could actually be beneficial as it prevents you from consuming food too close to bedtime. Although the "chewing phenomenon" wouldn't be relevant here, you would still be getting an adequate period of intermittent fasting while you sleep (for example, if you finish eating at 6 p.m. and then eat breakfast the next morning around 8 a.m., that's a total of 14 hours fasting, which is great). Again, we all have different habits and routines, and what works well for one person may not work at all for someone

KETO-FRIENDLY ALTERNATIVES

No matter what anyone says, there are *always* keto-friendly alternatives to high-carb foods. Yes, it may take some creativity, an open mind, and some habit changes, but it is most definitely doable.

Below is a chart of common foods and their keto alternatives that you can incorporate into your new lifestyle. Be sure to also check out my website, www.killinitketo.com, for more keto-friendly alternatives.

NOT SO FRIENDLY	KETO-FRIENDLY ALTERNATIVE
Biscuits, bread, rolls, wraps	Keto bread/rolls (Easy Keto Bread, page 241), lettuce wraps, low-carb tortillas, mushroom caps, Keto Biscuits (page 122)
Bread crumbs	Crushed pork rinds, grated cheese, almond flour, flaxseed meal, nutritional yeast
Chocolate and candy	Unsweetened cocoa/cacao, Mini Fat Bombs (page 247), Electrolyte Gummies (page 254)
Crackers and chips	Pork rinds, cheese crisps, kale chips, pepperoni/salami chips, Keto Crackers (page 136), crispy bacon, sliced vegetables, mixed nuts, dried seaweed
Milk and creamer	Heavy cream, unsweetened nut milks, unsweetened canned coconut milk/cream
Pasta	Zucchini noodles, shirataki noodles, shredded cabbage, spaghetti squash (in moderation)
Pizza crust	Omega-3 Pizza crust (page 167), chicken or other meat crust (Meatza Pizza, page 207), cauliflower crust
Potatoes (mashed or roasted) and French fries	Mashed cauliflower, roasted radishes, zucchini fries, avocado fries
Rice	Cauliflower rice, shirataki rice
Soda	Sparkling water, flavored electrolyte drinks, stevia-sweetened sodas like Zevia
Sugar	Stevia, monk fruit, erythritol
Wheat flour	Almond flour, coconut flour, collagen/protein powder, psyllium husk, or other nut/seed flours

else. Finding what works for *you* is the best way to be consistent and successful in the long run.

▶ Becoming Keto-Adapted

Transitioning from a sugar-burner to a fat-burner can take some time. Most of us have been running on carbohydrates and sugar our entire lives and our bodies have no idea what it feels like to truly be in "fat-burning mode."

There are a few different phases that our bodies go through during the adjustment period to becoming keto-adapted, and making sure you take the appropriate steps during each of these phases is crucial for long-term success. The exact length of each phase differs from person to person, but in general, following the steps outlined next will help you experience a smoother transition. During this challenge, you will transition through phase 1 and into phase 2. Phase 3 will come with time.

PHASE 1: GETTING INTO KETOSIS

Getting into a state of ketosis generally takes about two to three days for the average person. However, the transition can be difficult if you're not implementing the right tools. Make sure to follow these guidelines:

1. **Cut the carbs.** Reducing your carbohydrate intake is the first step toward producing ketones. Aim for 30 grams or less of total carbs per day and adjust accordingly.

2. **Consume enough *healthy* fats.** Throw your fear of fat out the window and fill your body with the exact fuel you want it to start using for energy—fat! This will ease the transition to becoming a more efficient fat-burner.

3. **Moderate protein.** Consuming too much protein, especially on its own, may spike insulin levels and make it harder to get into ketosis. Pair proteins with fats and be mindful of your intake.

4. **Replenish water and electrolytes.** When you reduce your carb intake, your body flushes out more water and takes sodium and other electrolytes with it. This can lead to symptoms of "keto flu," which is discussed in more detail on page 40.

5. **Avoid a severe caloric deficit.** Do not attempt to reduce your caloric intake during the first few days. Eat the same quantity of food that you normally eat while focusing on changing the macro composition: fewer carbs, moderate protein, more fat.

6. **Take it easy with exercise.** Cut back on the intensity and volume of exercise for the first few days (and maybe even during the first few weeks) to reduce the added stressors and promote a favorable transition. Focus on lighter activities like yoga and leisurely swims or walks.

PHASE 2: TRANSITIONING TO FAT-BURNING MODE

In phase 2, your body will start to transition to effectively using fat and ketones for fuel. This will lead to an increased feeling of fullness throughout the day, stable blood sugar levels, fewer cravings, endless energy, better mood, laser-sharp focus, and so much more. This phase generally begins at the end of the first week and will last for another six to eight weeks, depending on your adherence and prior metabolic health.

1. **Continue to replenish electrolytes.** Don't skimp on your electrolytes! It's important to continue replenishing these minerals (primarily sodium, magnesium, and potassium) every day, especially surrounding physical activity.

2. **Extend your fasting window.** Now that your blood sugar is beginning to stabilize and you're starting to feel more satiated during the day, try to reduce snacking, extend your morning fast, and/or shut the kitchen down earlier at night.

3. **Reduce caloric intake for fat loss.** As you become efficient at using fat and ketones for fuel while feeling more satiated during the day, you should naturally decrease the amount of food you're consuming. This will allow you

to start burning excess body fat. Use the guidelines on page 16 (Macro-nutrient Ratios for Weight Loss) as a starting place and adjust accordingly.

4. **Don't chase ketones.** If you regularly test ketones, you may start to see a reduction in your urine or blood levels. This is because your body and cells are starting to become more efficient at using fatty acids and ketones for fuel, which is a good thing! See page 42 for more details on testing ketones.

PHASE 3: BECOMING METABOLICALLY FLEXIBLE/EFFICIENT

This is essentially the phase that you want to get to and maintain for the remainder of your life. Becoming a full-on fat-burner is actually the normal, preferred state that humans are meant to thrive in. Once this is achieved, usually after four to six months or even up to a year, most people can effectively maintain a low-carbohydrate lifestyle while being able to incorporate healthy carb sources and enjoying occasional indulgences.

1. **Realize this is a lifestyle, not a diet.** If you look at keto as a diet, you will not succeed in the long term. If you go back to what you were doing before, you will end up exactly where you started.

2. **Experiment with small increases in protein and/or carbs.** After you've completely transitioned from a sugar-burner to a fat-burner, you can start to play around with your protein and carb threshold. Some people can bump up their carb and protein intake while still remaining in ketosis. This is highly individualized and takes some trial and error to figure out. People who have severe metabolic damage or who are trying to treat a disease state may not have this flexibility.

3. **Ease of going in and out of ketosis.** Now that you're a thriving fat-burner, your body will give you a bit more leeway when it comes to indulging in some carbs every once in a while. But don't use this as an excuse to go eat a whole carton of ice cream. Be strategic with your indulgences and don't get sidetracked when it comes to achieving and maintaining optimal health. Again, this is highly individualized and depends on your specific goals.

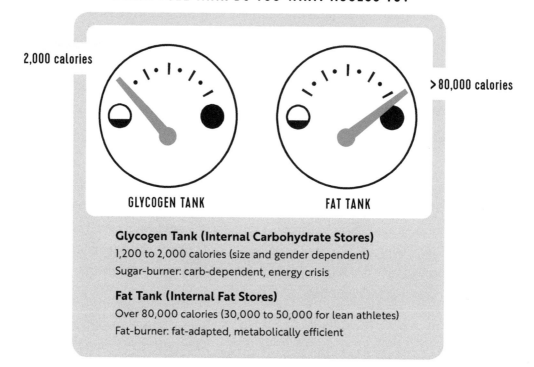

WHICH FUEL TANK DO YOU WANT ACCESS TO?

2,000 calories

>80,000 calories

GLYCOGEN TANK

FAT TANK

Glycogen Tank (Internal Carbohydrate Stores)
1,200 to 2,000 calories (size and gender dependent)
Sugar-burner: carb-dependent, energy crisis

Fat Tank (Internal Fat Stores)
Over 80,000 calories (30,000 to 50,000 for lean athletes)
Fat-burner: fat-adapted, metabolically efficient

THE KETO FLU

When transitioning into phase 1 of keto-adaptation, you may experience initial side effects, known as "keto flu," that come with cutting carbs. These side effects include headaches, brain fog, irritability, nausea, dizziness, muscle cramps, heart palpitations, insomnia, diarrhea, fatigue, weakness, and carb cravings. If you're highly dependent on carbs and processed foods for energy, you may experience worse symptoms than someone who is more accustomed to a lower-carb diet. However, the main culprit of the keto flu is usually an improper balance and deficiency of necessary electrolytes—primarily sodium, potassium, and magnesium.

When you reduce your carb intake, your body begins to excrete more water. This is because carbs hold on to water in your body, and as your insulin levels drop, your kidneys are triggered to excrete more water. As water goes, it takes electrolytes with it. Combatting the keto flu is actually pretty easy if you implement the guidelines in phase 1 and make sure to adequately replenish your water and electrolyte intake. You should aim for the following daily amounts:

Water: Consume *at least* half your body weight in ounces per day (more if you work out and sweat heavily). For example, if you weigh 190 pounds, you should consume at least 95 ounces (190/2 = 95) of water per day. In general, drinking at least eight 8-ounce glasses of water a day is a good place to start.

Sodium: Aim for 4,000 to 6,000 milligrams per day (about 2 to 2½ teaspoons of salt).

- Do not be afraid of salt! It is your friend when following a ketogenic protocol.
- Add sea salt—in the form of pink salt or Celtic sea salt—to your food or drinks each day (especially surrounding physical activity).
- Drink Bone Broth (page 240).
- Consume salty foods like pickles, bacon, salted nuts, seeds, etc.

Potassium: Aim for 3,000 to 4,000 milligrams per day.

- Eat potassium-rich foods (see sidebar on page 43).
- Supplement options:
  - Cream of tartar: ½ teaspoon = 250 mg of potassium
  - Potassium chloride and potassium citrate are in several popular electrolyte powder drinks, brands like Lite Salt or NoSalt (sodium + potassium), or in pill or capsule form.

Magnesium: Aim for 400 to 800 milligrams per day.

- Eat magnesium-rich foods (see sidebar on page 43).
- Supplement with high-quality, chelated magnesium. Some popular, absorbable forms include (but are not limited to):
  - Magnesium glycinate—shown to have high absorption rate, calming, and may help with nerve pain.
  - Magnesium L-threonate—may help with brain cognition and function.

- Magnesium citrate—budget-friendly option but may cause loose stools (could help with constipation).
- Magnesium sulfate (also known as Epsom salt)—helps soothe muscles and supports relaxation.
- Tips:
  - Magnesium helps you relax and certain forms are best taken before bed.
  - Avoid magnesium oxide—a non-absorbable form of magnesium and strong laxative.

If you're very active, consider supplementing with electrolytes surrounding your workouts or enjoy a Keto Flu Combat Smoothie (page 114).

- Popular electrolyte drink powders:
  - Ultima Replenisher
  - Vega Sport Electrolyte Hydrator
  - Zipfizz
- Popular electrolyte supplements:
  - Keto Vitals
  - Perfect Keto Electrolytes

▶ Testing Your Ketones

Ketones are produced when your body breaks down fat for energy. There are three different types of ketone bodies: acetoacetate, acetone, and beta-hydroxybutyrate (BHB), and there are different ways to test each.

Testing Your Urine (tests for acetoacetate):

Pros: Cheap, quick, and useful if you're just starting keto to see if you're beginning to produce ketones.

Cons: Not reliable, especially after a few weeks. Hydration status can affect results.

Using ketone urine strips is the least accurate method of testing because it actually measures the amount of ketones that your body is excreting, instead of

Sodium	Celtic sea salt, Himalayan sea salt, Bone Broth (page 240), fermented vegetables, cured meats
Magnesium	Spinach, Swiss chard, nuts, pumpkin seeds, artichokes, unsweetened cacao/cocoa powder, unsweetened chocolate, fish
Potassium	Meats, beet and radish leaves, avocados, dark leafy greens, dried herbs, zucchini, salmon, sardines, mushrooms, nuts, cream of tartar, cacao/cocoa powder, unsweetened chocolate
Calcium	Cheeses, green vegetables, sardines, almonds, kefir
Phosphorus	Meats, eggs, cheeses, nuts, seeds, fish, unsweetened chocolate
Chloride	Olives, seaweed, vegetables, salt (sodium chloride)

using for fuel. It's common to see high levels of urine ketones when first starting a ketogenic diet because your body isn't efficient at using ketones for energy yet, so they are wasted through urine. As you become more adapted and efficient at using ketones for fuel, the amount excreted through urine will naturally decrease.

Testing Your Breath (tests for acetone, which is a byproduct from the breakdown of acetoacetate):

Pros: Cost effective in the long term, reusable device, reliable for testing acetone, easy to use.

Cons: Doesn't correlate directly with blood ketone levels. Alcohol consumption can cause a false-positive reading. Water intake and other factors like gum chewing or mouthwash can affect results.

Breath ketone monitors can give you a good idea of how much fat your body is turning into fuel, but it doesn't necessarily correlate with the amount of BHB in your blood, which is currently the most accurate measure of testing. Common devices on the market right now are the Ketonix Breath Analyzer and the LEVL Breath Ketone Meter.

Testing Your Blood (tests for beta-hydroxybutyrate or BHB):

Pros: Most reliable and accurate measurement.

Cons: Expensive, requires a needle finger prick for blood.

Blood ketone testing is currently considered the gold standard for measuring ketone levels. Nutritional ketosis is traditionally defined as having a blood ketone range between 0.5 and 5.0 mmol/L. Time of day and exercise can affect levels, so stay consistent when testing. MCT oil/powder or other forms of fat may throw off the accuracy of your results, so try not to consume them before testing. Common devices include the Precision Xtra Blood Glucose & Ketone Monitoring System from Abbott and the Keto-Mojo Ketone and Blood Glucose Monitoring System.

A few notes on testing ketones:

- Testing ketones is not completely necessary, but it can be helpful, especially when first embarking on your keto journey.
- Higher ketone levels *do not* equal more weight loss. Don't chase ketones, chase results!
- Alternative signs that can still be an accurate way of detecting if you're becoming keto-adapted and using fat for fuel:
  - Fruity breath or a sour, metallic taste in your mouth (usually subsides after the first week or two and doesn't occur in everyone).
  - Enhanced focus, mental clarity, and increased or steady energy throughout the day with no afternoon crash.
  - Reduced hunger, lack of cravings, and ability to go longer periods of time without eating.
  - An overall feeling of calmness and stabilized mood.

If you're a diabetic, whether type 1 or 2, you can most definitely benefit from adopting a low-carbohydrate, ketogenic lifestyle. For those with type 1 diabetes, this lifestyle can greatly improve blood sugar control; for type 2 diabetics, it can aid in reducing medications and ultimately lead to reversal of the condition. Recently, one of my colleagues, Dr. Brian Lenzkes, an internal medicine physician, has successfully taken more than 10 of his type 2 diabetic patients off insulin in just a matter of six months.

That being said, it's extremely important that you consult with your doctor before embarking on this journey so that you can effectively manage medications and properly monitor blood glucose levels and insulin dosages. This is especially important for those with type 1 diabetes or severe type 2 diabetes, to prevent any risk of diabetic ketoacidosis.

Diabetic ketoacidosis is completely different from nutritional ketosis, which is one of the major misconceptions that doctors and other people can have.

- **Diabetic ketoacidosis** is a toxic metabolic state that occurs when there is uncontrolled ketone production (greater than 15 mmol/L), high concentrations of blood glucose, and an increase in the acidity of blood (or lowered blood pH).

- **Nutritional ketosis** is a normal metabolic state that occurs when the production of ketones does not generally exceed 7 to 8 mmol/L, blood glucose levels are normal and stabilized, and there is no change in blood acidity (or pH levels).

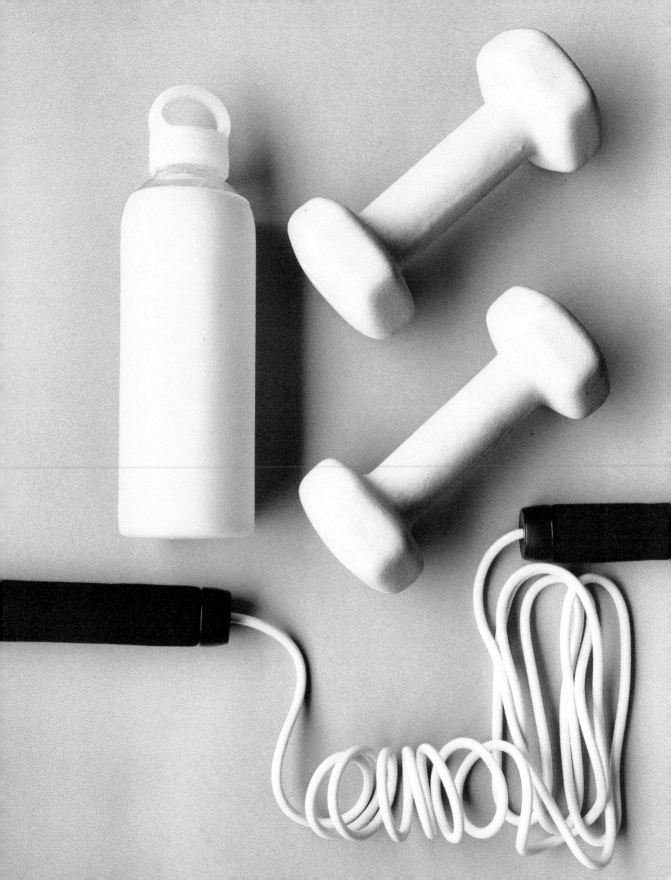

3

Exercise, Sleep, Stress Management, and Mind-set

The second pillar of your keto challenge is exercise. Although exercise is vital for overall health and wellness, I believe that diet, sleep, stress management, and mind-set play a larger role when it comes to a successful weight-loss program. The "eat less, exercise more" approach may work in the beginning, but it is not sustainable and has been shown to cause more harm than good in the long term. That being said, if you can incorporate an exercise routine that is enjoyable, sustainable, and boosts your mental well-being, you may reach your goals faster, setting you on the right path to a healthier and more active lifestyle.

The final pillars of your keto challenge—sleep, stress management, and mind-set—are too often overlooked when embarking on a challenge like this. So often, people come to me saying they're following the diet to a tee, exercising all the time, and still not seeing results. But it turns out they are sleeping only four or five hours a night, stressed out at work, and forgetting why they even embarked on this lifestyle. These factors can have a huge impact on your weight-loss efforts.

This chapter provides several tips and strategies for how to develop a sustainable exercise program, balance your sleep, reduce stress, and adopt a mind-set that will help you achieve lasting weight loss and an overall healthier lifestyle.

▶ Setting an Exercise Routine

If you are starting this challenge with an exercise routine that you already currently enjoy and feel is sustainable, then by all means continue with that routine. If you have never exercised before or feel intimidated by the thought of starting, don't worry; the recommendations in this chapter are based on a gradual progression to help you build a plan that works for your lifestyle.

Ideally, exercise should include a combination of both strength-training and aerobic (cardio) activities to help build strong muscles and bones, increase the efficiency of your heart and lungs, and improve other important components such as mood, hormonal activity, and overall energy. In the following section, we will cover different types of exercise, the benefits of each, and various examples that you can begin incorporating into your own exercise regimen.

STRENGTH TRAINING

Strength training, in my opinion, is the most important form of exercise a person can do. Not only does it build a strong foundation for every form of physical activity, it also sets your body up to burn more energy (calories) at rest and thus can enhance weight loss. These are some of the many benefits associated with strength training:

Increased muscle mass and tone. That means more energy (calories) burned throughout the day.

Strengthened bones, connective tissue, tendons, and core. These help maintain balance and mobility and decrease risk of injuries.

Improved sense of well-being. This boosts mood, self-confidence, and overall feelings of happiness.

Enhanced performance of everyday tasks. You'll have greater stamina and the ability to perform everyday tasks more efficiently.

Here are a few examples of different strength-training modalities that you can include in your exercise routine.

Free weights include dumbbells, barbells, kettle bells, medicine balls, or really anything that can be held and used as a weight.

Weight machines are found in classic gyms and usually focus more on individual muscle groups and isolation exercises.

Body weight exercises include squats, push-ups, pull-ups, lunges, planks, and other core exercises.

Resistance bands provide continuous resistance throughout a movement and are portable, inexpensive, and adaptable for any fitness level.

CARDIOVASCULAR EXERCISE

Cardiovascular exercise, or aerobic training, is important for improving heart and lung function, increasing circulation, and, more specific to the ketogenic lifestyle, enhancing your ability to burn fat efficiently. Cardiovascular exercise has the following benefits:

Increased size and number of mitochondria. Mitochondria are the energy-producing cells in your body where fat is burned. More mitochondria means more fat-burning potential.

Strengthened heart and lungs. Performing cardio exercises increases heart rate and forces your lungs to work harder and thus get stronger.

Reduced stress and anxiety. Cardio leads to the release of endorphins, also known as the "feel-good" hormone.

There are many different types of cardio exercise out there, and it really comes down to choosing the ones that you enjoy the most. Some of the more common ones include:

- Walking
- Jogging
- Running
- Biking
- Swimming
- Hiking
- Rowing
- Elliptical
- Stair climbing

INTERVAL TRAINING

Interval training is a form of cardiovascular exercise that focuses on alternating between high- and low-intensity exercise. It includes incorporating short bursts of "all-out" work followed by less intense recovery periods and repeating this for a set period of time. Interval training stimulates your metabolism to burn lots of calories not only during the workout, but also for an extended period after the workout is complete. There are many benefits to interval training:

Saves time and decreases boredom. Typical interval workouts only last between 10 and 20 minutes, making them efficient and more appealing.

Increases fat-burning potential. Short, high-intensity workouts stimulate the release of human growth hormone (HGH), also known as the "fat-burning hormone."

Boosts post-exercise calorie burn. Interval training stimulates your body to burn calories for a longer period of time following the workout.

The cool thing about interval training is that it can be done using any type of exercise listed. Just pick the one you enjoy the most and implement it into one of the protocols listed below. Always warm up first, cool down after, and increase the intensity as you become more comfortable.

HIIT (High-Intensity Interval Training):

- A short, intense bout of exercise followed by a set period of rest.

- Examples of a 10- to 15-minute HIIT workout progression:

    - **Week 1:** 10 seconds on, 30 seconds off

    - **Week 2:** 20 seconds on, 45 seconds off

    - **Week 3:** 30 seconds on, 30 seconds off

    - **Week 4:** 1 minute on, 1 minute off

    - **Week 5:** 1 minute on, 30 seconds off

- Increase intensity and time, decrease rest period as you become more adapted.

Tabata—another popular form of HIIT:

- Warm up for 5 to 10 minutes.

- Perform 20 seconds of all-out, high-intensity work, followed by 10 seconds rest. Repeat for a total of 8 rounds (4 minutes total).

- Cool down for 5 to 10 minutes.

- Repeat with different modalities and increase intensity as you adapt.

These are just a few examples of how you can build an HIIT routine. There are many different combinations and variations of exercises you can incorporate, and these will also depend on your specific goals and modalities of choice.

CIRCUIT TRAINING

Circuit training is essentially a combination of cardio and strength training with a similar foundation to interval training. It involves a fast-paced workout using different forms of resistance exercises with little to no rest between movements. Circuit training is my favorite because you get the benefits of cardio, strength, and interval training all wrapped up into one 20- to 30-minute exercise session. It's quick, effective, and the possibilities to mix things up are endless.

You can easily build your own circuit-training workout by following these guidelines:

1. **Choose your time limit.** Typical circuits last anywhere from 10 to 45 minutes. The shorter the workout, the harder you should be working during each exercise.

2. **Pick a lower body exercise.** Use whatever you have on hand or just use your body weight. Feel free to switch up the movement each round or stick with the same one throughout the entire workout to keep it simple.

   Examples:
   - Squats
   - Lunges
   - Step-ups
   - Wall sits

3. **Pick an upper body exercise.** Follow the same guidelines as for the lower body exercise.

Examples:
- Push-ups
- Bent-over rows
- Shoulder press
- Triceps dip
- Bicep curls

4. **Pick a compound or full-body exercise.** Compound or multi-joint movements stimulate more muscles at once and get your heart rate up.

Examples:
- Burpees
- Mountain climbers
- Jumping lunges
- Thrusters (squat to shoulder press)

5. **Choose a sprint exercise.** Pick a cardio exercise and go all out for 30 seconds to 1 minute.

Examples:
- Running
- Rowing
- Jumping rope
- Jumping jacks
- Biking
- Stair climbing

6. **Rest and repeat.** Rest for about 1 minute and then go back through the circuit as many times as you can within your allotted time frame.

▶ Exercise Myths

There is too much misinformation these days about exercise and how it pertains to weight loss and the ketogenic lifestyle. Many people fall short of their goals because of bogus information. Let's dispel a few of these myths.

Myth: You need carbohydrates to fuel your workouts. Our bodies store over 40,000 calories of fat and only about 2,000 calories of carbs. Becoming fat-adapted allows you access to endless amounts of energy for fuel and increases metabolic flexibility (the ability to switch from one fuel source to another). Plus, carbs are not essential for survival—fat and protein are!

Myth: You need to exercise to lose weight. Successful and sustainable weight loss occurs with proper diet and lifestyle. Hormonal balance, stress levels, sleep, and positive mind-set are far more important for weight loss. Exercise can help, but it is only a small piece of the puzzle.

Myth: More time means more calories burned. Exercising for 10 to 20 minutes at a high intensity, or strength training to build muscle, will burn way more calories than walking on the treadmill for an hour. This is mostly due to the *afterburn* effect that comes with high-intensity and strength-training routines.

Myth: Lifting heavy weights makes women bulky. Lifting heavy weights stimulates more muscle growth. More muscle means more fat-burning potential and a leaner and more defined physique. Plus, women don't produce enough testosterone to "bulk up" like men do. Lift heavy when you can.

▶ Getting the Most Out of Your Workouts

Fitting exercise into your daily schedule may seem difficult or overwhelming at first. Here are some tips for getting the most out of your workouts:

Find something you love. The best way to start incorporating exercise into your lifestyle is to find something that you enjoy doing. Choose an activity that excites you and you will be much more likely to actually do it.

Set a goal and challenge yourself. Setting a specific goal makes it much easier to find motivation and stick with a routine. If you don't have a specific reason for doing something, you probably won't do it. Set a goal that inspires you and challenge yourself each week to work toward it.

Get competitive. Just like goal setting, having some competition involved can really boost your drive to get after it. Whether that's signing up for some type of race or competition, creating weekly challenges with your family and friends, or joining a group exercise class such as CrossFit. You'll be surprised how fun and rewarding it is to partake in some friendly competition.

Keep it short and intense. Don't waste your valuable time wandering around the gym or walking on a treadmill for hours. Incorporate interval or circuit training and get a more efficient and effective workout in as little as 10 minutes.

Switch things up. If you start getting bored with your routine, change it up. This helps both mentally and physically by keeping your mind, body, and muscles guessing.

▶ Recommendations

When starting a ketogenic protocol, it is important to realize that your energy levels and ability to exert yourself will probably be minimal during the first few days and up to a week for some people. This is completely normal and occurs because your body is in the process of switching its primary fuel source from carbs and sugar to fat and ketones.

I have found that backing off from physical activity during the first week or two helps most people transition more smoothly and with the fewest negative side effects. That being said, if you're a regular exerciser and want to continue with your daily regimen, by all means do so. Just make sure you replenish your electrolytes sufficiently and give your body a break if it is not performing to your typical standards.

The primary goal of this 21-day challenge is to get your keto diet protocol right. This is important to understand because I have seen many people embark on both a completely new diet regimen and a new workout routine at the same time, leading to unnecessary stress, feeling totally overwhelmed, and ultimately giving up before they can experience any of the amazing benefits.

So, during this challenge, I am going to suggest weekly workout plans that evolve gradually as you become adapted. The idea is to get your body moving from the start but without adding too much mental and physical stress. The ultimate goal is for you to find an effective and enjoyable workout routine that fits your lifestyle and helps you reach your individual goals.

GO-TO EXERCISE CIRCUITS

Next you'll find three simple, quick, yet effective exercise circuits that can easily be done at home or when traveling. Remember to always warm up for 5 to 10 minutes before beginning any workout. This can include jogging in place for a few minutes or going through one round of the circuit at a slow, warm-up pace.

Use the following categories to choose your exercises for each circuit (detailed descriptions of each exercise are on pages 57–63):

1. **Full body** (jumping jack, burpee, mountain climber)

2. **Upper body** (push-up, bent-over rows, triceps dip, shoulder press)

3. **Lower body** (squat, lunge, wall sit, glute bridge)

4. **Core** (plank, bicycle crunch, hollow rock)

Circuit 1: Traditional Strength Circuit

Choose one exercise from each category and perform 2 or 3 rounds of 8 to 10 repetitions per exercise. Mix up the exercises when performing them on different days of the week.

Sample Circuit 1

1. **Burpees** (full body): Perform 2 or 3 sets of 8 to 10 repetitions per set.

2. **Bent-over rows** (upper body): Perform 2 or 3 sets of 8 to 10 repetitions per set.

3. **Squats** (lower body): Perform 2 or 3 sets of 8 to 10 repetitions per set.

4. **Hollow rock** (core): Perform 2 or 3 sets of 8 to 10 repetitions per set.

Circuit 2: Work, Rest, Repeat

Choose one exercise from each category. Perform each exercise for 30 seconds and then rest for 10 seconds as you transition to the next exercise. Repeat 2 or 3 times. As you progress, increase the intensity, duration, or number of sets.

Tip: Download an Interval Timer application on your phone for an easy way to track your work and rest periods.

1. **Mountain Climbers** (full body): Perform as many mountain climbers as you can in 30 seconds. Rest for 10 seconds and move on to the next exercise.

2. **Triceps dips** (upper body): Perform as many triceps dips as you can in 30 seconds. Rest for 10 seconds and move on to the next exercise.

3. **Lunges** (lower body): Perform as many alternating lunges as you can in 30 seconds. Rest for 10 seconds and move on to the next exercise.

4. **Plank** (core): Perform a 30-second plank hold. Rest for 10 seconds and return to exercise #1.

Circuit 3: Descending Ladder

Choose one exercise from each category. Perform 10 repetitions (reps) of the first category exercise, followed by 10 reps of the second category exercise. Then perform 9 reps of the first category exercise, followed by 9 reps of the second category exercise. Continue the descending ladder until you finish with 1 rep of each.

Sample Circuit 3: Upper and Lower Body Ladder

10 push-ups, 10 squats, 9 push-ups, 9 squats, 8 push-ups, 8 squats . . . 2 push-ups, 2 squats, 1 push-up, 1 squat.

Sample Circuit 3: Full Body and Core Ladder

10 burpees, 10 hollow rocks, 9 burpees, 9 hollow rocks, 8 burpees, 8 hollow rocks . . . 2 burpees, 2 hollow rocks, 1 burpee, 1 hollow rock.

EXERCISE DEMONSTRATIONS

Full Body

JUMPING JACK

Start by standing with your feet together, knees slightly bent, and arms down by your sides. Brace your abs and jump both legs out to the side, landing with your feet just wider than your hips and raising your arms overhead. Keep your knees slightly bent while you jump again to bring your feet back together and your arms down to your side. This counts as one repetition.

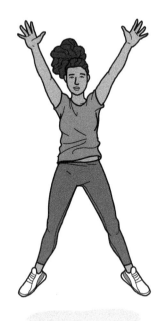

BURPEE

Start by standing with your feet hip-width apart. Lower yourself into a squat. Place your hands on the floor in front of you and shift your weight forward. Jump or walk your feet back into a plank position, keeping your abs braced, making sure your body creates a straight line. Jump or walk your feet back toward your hands and return to the bottom of the squat. Jump or stand up, reaching your arms straight overhead. This constitutes one repetition.

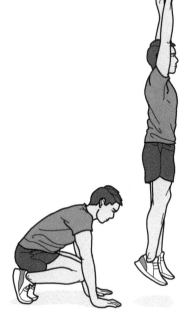

MOUNTAIN CLIMBER

Start on the floor in a push-up position. Maintain a slight arch in your back and raise one knee toward your chest. Pause, return to the starting position, and repeat with your other leg. This constitutes one repetition. Alternate until you have completed all your reps.

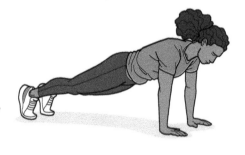
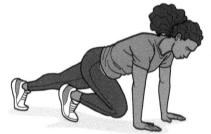

Upper Body

PUSH-UP

Start on the floor with your hands directly under your shoulders. Lift your body into a plank position with your weight evenly distributed on your hands and feet. Draw your shoulder blades back and down your back, while keeping your elbows close to your body. Lower your body until your chest touches the floor. Make sure your abs and glutes are still engaged and exhale as you push yourself up, in one straight line, to the starting position. If this is too challenging, keep your knees on the floor while performing the push-up.

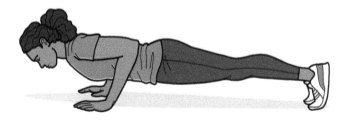

BENT-OVER ROWS

Start by standing with your feet hip-width apart. Hold a dumbbell in each hand, palms facing each other. Bend your knees slightly and bring your chest forward by bending at your waist. As you bend, make sure to keep your back straight until it is almost parallel to the floor. Brace your abs and lift the dumbbells to your sides, keeping your elbows close to your body. Squeeze your back muscles at the top, hold for a second, and then slowly lower the weights to the starting position. This counts as one repetition.

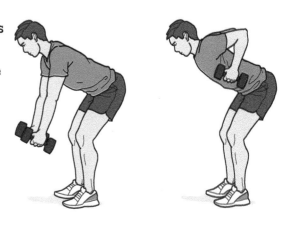

TRICEPS DIP

Start by sitting on the floor in front of a step, bench, or sturdy chair. With your knees slightly bent and feet planted firmly on the floor, grab the edge of the elevated surface behind you, and place your hands slightly wider than shoulder-width apart. Bend your arms to a 90-degree angle, keeping your elbows close to your body. Brace your abs and straighten your arms, pushing through your heels. Lower back down to a seated position. This counts as one repetition.

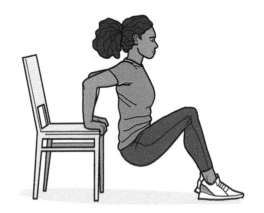

SHOULDER PRESS

Start by standing with your feet hip-width apart and a dumbbell (or other sturdy weight) in each hand. Raise the weights to shoulder height and bring your elbows to a 90-degree angle. Brace your abs and extend through your elbows to raise the weights together directly above your head. Pause at the top and then slowly return to the starting position.

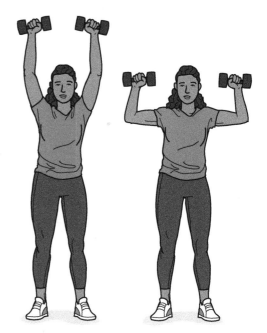

Lower Body

SQUAT

Start by standing with your feet hip-width apart or slightly wider. Extend your hands straight out in front of you for balance. Brace your abs and sit back and down like you're sitting into an imaginary chair. Keep your chest up and look straight ahead. Go as far down as you can without dropping your chest. Once you reach your depth, press through your heels and spring back into the standing position, squeezing your glutes at the top. This counts as one repetition.

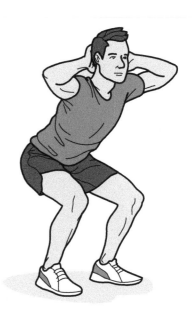

LUNGE

Start by standing with your feet a bit wider than hip-width apart. Brace your abs and take a big step forward with your left foot. Make sure your knees, hips, and shoulders all face forward. Keep your chest up, brace your abs, and sink straight down until your left knee makes a 90-degree angle and your right knee is pointing straight down toward the floor. Ensure your left knee does not go past your toes. Shift the weight onto the ball of your right foot as you push back up, and step back into the starting position. This counts as one repetition.

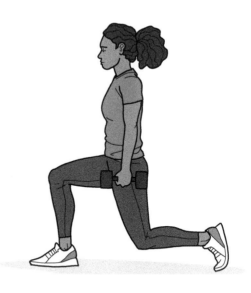

WALL SIT

Start by standing with your back against a wall. Slowly slide down the wall until your thighs are parallel to the ground, making a 90-degree angle. Make sure your knees are directly above your ankles, keep your back straight, and hold your arms straight out in front of you. Hold the position for 8 to 10 seconds. This counts as one repetition.

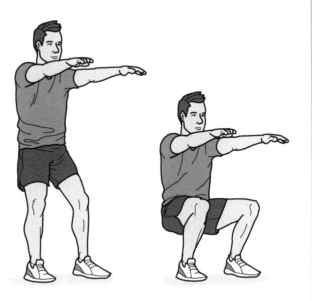

GLUTE BRIDGE

Start by lying on your back on the floor with your hands by your sides and your knees bent. Your feet should be hip-width apart. With your weight in your heels, breathe out as you lift your hips off the floor while keeping your back straight. Hold at the top for a few seconds and then slowly lower back to the floor as you breathe in.

Variation: Perform the exercise on one leg at a time with the other leg straight in the air.

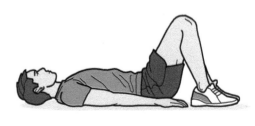

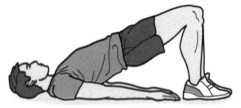

Core

PLANK

Start on your stomach on the floor. Place your forearms on the floor with your elbows aligned directly under your shoulders, forming a 90-degree angle. Raise your knees off the ground, supporting your weight on your toes and forearms. Your body should form a straight line from your head to your feet. Set your gaze at a point on the floor about a foot in front of you, and make sure your neck is in line with the rest of your body. Breathe as you hold this position, squeezing your core and glutes, for the allotted time period.

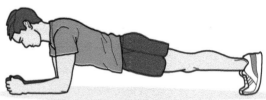

BICYCLE CRUNCH

Start by lying on your back on the floor. Bring your knees to your chest and place your hands behind your head, interlocking your fingers. Lift your shoulders off the floor, tighten your abs, and tuck your chin into your chest. Touch the inside of your right arm to the inside of your left thigh while straightening your right leg. Alternate and touch the inside of your left arm to the inside of your right thigh while straightening your left leg. This counts as one repetition.

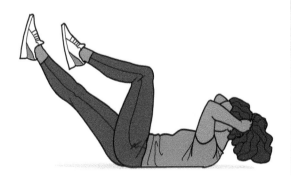

HOLLOW ROCK

Start by lying on your back on the floor. Contract your abs while pressing your lower back into the floor. With your legs straight and toes pointed, raise your legs off the floor a couple of inches. Straighten your arms above your head and raise them off the floor so they are aligned with your ears. Keeping your lower back on the floor and abs engaged, rock back and forth without allowing the shape to break. This counts as one repetition.

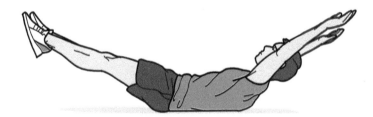

▶ Sleep

Lack of sleep is one of the easiest ways to throw off hormonal balance and prevent you from losing weight. This leads to issues like insulin resistance (talked about in more detail in chapter 1), impaired functioning of leptin and ghrelin, hormones that control a large portion of hunger and satiety, and chronic elevations of cortisol, the hormone associated with stress. When these hormones are not functioning properly it makes losing weight and keeping it off nearly impossible.

Rather than just tell you that you need between seven and nine hours of sleep each night, I'm going to provide you with some tips on how to achieve quality, restful sleep that will help balance your hormones and turn you into a fat-burning machine.

BEST PRACTICES FOR RESTFUL SLEEP

Create the optimal bedroom. A cool, quiet, dark, and comfortable environment is essential for achieving quality sleep.

- Keep the temperature between 60°F and 70°F and make sure your bedroom is well ventilated.

- Reduce outside noise by using earplugs or a peaceful white noise machine or fan.

- Use blackout curtains or an eye mask to block light.

- Invest in a good quality mattress and consider using a weighted blanket if you're prone to experiencing sleep anxiety.

- Keep electronics—TV, cell phone, computer—out of the bedroom to decrease distraction and avoid exposure to blue light.

Keep your circadian rhythm in check. Properly regulating your body's internal clock, also known as the circadian rhythm, is extremely important for promoting restful sleep. Here are a few tips for keeping your circadian rhythm functioning optimally.

- Increase exposure to natural light during the day by taking a morning walk or lunchtime stroll. Natural light helps reset your biological clock and balances hormones associated with sleep, such as serotonin and melatonin.

- Exercise earlier in the day to prevent a surge of cortisol at the wrong time. Cortisol is a hormone that is naturally high in the morning and should fall throughout the day. If you exercise too close to bedtime, it can disrupt your natural ability to wind down and fall asleep.

- Avoid exposure to artificial light at night. Bright lights in the evening can throw off your circadian clock by confusing your brain into thinking it's daytime. Artificial blue light coming from your cell phone, TV, or computer inhibits your body's natural production of melatonin, the sleepy-time hormone. Reduce exposure by wearing blue blocking glasses (inexpensive and easily available on Amazon), turning your cell phone to "night time mode," and/or shutting down the electronics and reading a book as it gets closer to bedtime.

- Maintain a regular sleep schedule so your body gets used to going to bed and waking up at the same time each day, making it easier to fall asleep and wake up naturally.

These are just a few of the natural strategies you can implement to help increase quality sleep and balance hormones throughout the day and night. A few others that I've found helpful include:

- Limiting caffeine consumption after 1 p.m.

- Taking a magnesium supplement (see Keto Flu, page 40)

- Sipping hot, caffeine-free tea

▶ Stress Management

We all face different stressors each day, whether it's the good stress that comes from a hard exercise session or the bad, chronic stress that stems from an unhealthy relationship or unpleasant work environment. Stress is everywhere, and finding ways to effectively manage it is a major key to finding short-term, and more importantly, long-term success with this program.

Embarking on this challenge is a stressor in itself, so let's discuss specific strategies that can help minimize some of the other stressors in your life and ease the transition to this healthier lifestyle.

BEST PRACTICES FOR STRESS MANAGEMENT

Plan ahead. Not only is planning ahead crucial for success, it's also the key to reducing the mental and emotional fatigue that comes along with the stress of not being prepared. Prep your meals and plan your exercise routine at the beginning of the week, keep daily checklists, and set deadlines for specifics tasks you'd like to complete.

Learn how to relax. Whether it's watching TV, reading a book, doing yoga, or taking a hot bath, finding ways to implement relaxation in your daily routine plays a huge role in reducing stress levels.

Get moving . . . but be smart about it. My personal favorite way to destress is going to the gym or listening to a podcast while taking a long walk during my lunch break. Movement and physical activity naturally reduce stress by helping release the "feel-good" hormones in your body. But be mindful, too much exercise or taking part in exercise that you don't enjoy can add unnecessary stress.

Increase your social support. Find people who have similar interests or goals. Having a support system not only helps with daily motivation and adherence, but also gives you somewhere to turn for help or reassurance when things get tough. My online program has a private Facebook group where participants share their daily struggles and successes to help teach and motivate each other.

Try meditating. Practicing meditation can help your mind and body become relaxed and focused, letting you release built-up emotions and increase self-awareness, among many other things. Even just five minutes a day of meditation can have a huge impact on stress reduction. If you've never meditated before, start with a guided meditation. There are several phone applications that are free to download and use.

Practice gratitude. Reflecting on what you are grateful for in your life can lead to an immense amount of positive emotion and overall stress reduction. Simply set a daily morning or evening routine and write down three things you are grateful for and why. Creating a daily gratitude habit could be just the thing to get those positive juices flowing and help you become more aware of all the good in your life.

▶ Mind-set

It's easy to come up with a plan, set a goal, and tell yourself you're going to follow through with it. The hard part is *actually* following through. Here's the thing . . . the diet and exercise part is not what makes this challenge a challenge, it's the way you approach the challenge mentally and emotionally that will determine your success. And I'm not just talking about a sudden light switch going off in your head telling you "okay, it's time to lose weight." It's more than that.

Getting your mind right takes a bit of work, and for true long-term success, you have to learn how to shift your mind-set to a more positive and realistic state. In this section, we are going to look at the ways that mind-set can both help us and harm us. We're going to discuss strategies to avoid falling into the traps of negative thinking and self-judgment, while also finding ways to reverse bad habits and stay motivated, not just during this challenge but throughout the rest of your journey.

MAKE A COMMITMENT

Making a commitment involves dedicating yourself to something and is the first step to getting your mind on the right track. By reading this book, you are making a commitment to your health and prioritizing self-care. You've made the commitment and now it's time to take action.

SET GOALS

We've all been taught that setting goals is an important part of life because it helps us have a long-term vision while keeping short-term motivation strong. It sounds cliché, but setting goals *is* extremely important; it keeps you focused, allows you to measure progress, and helps bust through distractions and procrastination.

But it's important to realize that goal setting only works when it is done in a realistic and straightforward manner. If you try to set goals that are impractical or overly complex, you will fall short and risk losing motivation. The following is a reliable and practical method to help you create your goals.

Step #1: Create goals that excite and motivate you

Rather than just focusing on the main goal of weight loss, think about specific reasons why losing weight will help you achieve other goals—whether that's playing outside with your kids without getting out of breath or planning a vacation with friends where you can put on a bathing suit and actually feel comfortable in your own skin. Making sure the goal is important to you and puts a smile on your face when you think about the successful outcome increases the likelihood of you putting in the work to make it happen.

Step #2: Set SMART goals

This SMART goals checklist will help you clarify your ideas, focus your efforts, and increase your chances of success. Consider whether your goal to lose weight fits the following criteria.

Specific. Your goal must be clear and specific. Rather than setting a general goal to lose weight, focus on a milestone or accomplishment you'd like to reach that brings you closer to achieving weight loss. For example, set a goal to stop snacking at night, or to push your first meal of the day to a few hours later. The more specific you are, the better motivated you will be.

Measurable. Your goal must be measurable so you can track your progress, meet your deadline, and feel the excitement building as you get closer to achieving it. For example, keep a journal and write down what time you ate your last bite of food at night or took the first bite in the morning. This will help you keep track of how well you are sticking to this specific goal.

Attainable. Your goal needs to be realistic and achievable. It should challenge you to some extent but not be impossible to follow through with each day. Answer the question: "How can I accomplish this goal?" For example, if your goal is to stop snacking at night, one way to accomplish it is to replace the snackless void with something else, such as drinking a cup of tea, taking a hot bath, or taking part in a nighttime yoga session.

Relevant. Your goal must matter and should fit within the bigger picture of what you're trying to accomplish. Cutting back on nighttime snacking prevents you from consuming unnecessary calories and can help you adopt new and better habits that will further your success in the long term.

Time bound. Every goal needs to have a deadline for you to work toward and stay focused as you progress. Create a timeframe that keeps you accountable. For example, give yourself three weeks to change your nighttime snacking habit. Maybe the first week you shut the kitchen down at 9 p.m., the second week at 8 p.m., and the third week at 7 p.m.

Step #3: Write your goals down

Dust off that notebook and take 10 minutes to actually write down your goals using the SMART goal checklist. A good method is to start by writing down one long-term goal and three short-term goals, moving through the SMART goal checklist for each one. Make sure to use "will" instead of "might" or "would like to."

This increases your power to achieve that goal, knowing that it's something you *will* stick to. Writing your goals down makes them real, and posting them in visible places such as on your refrigerator, desk, or mirror helps keep you accountable and prevents an "out of sight, out of mind" mentality.

You can set all the goals you want, but if you don't plan and take action to achieve them, you will have wasted your time. Write out the individual steps you will take to achieve each goal and then check each one off as you complete it. This visual confirmation of your progress will encourage you and keep your mind focused and on the right track for long-term success.

IDENTIFY BAD HABITS

Recognizing and being mindful of your own bad habits can help prevent you falling into some of the same traps that have kept you from hitting weight-loss goals in the past. We are all creatures of habit, and exchanging bad habits for good ones doesn't happen overnight. It takes gradual action steps and continuous patterns to reverse and replace bad habits with better ones. Here are a few common habits that I see often:

Snacking at night or when bored. This is one that I've always personally struggled with. The routine of having dessert after dinner or sitting in front of the TV with something to munch on is extremely hard to break. Rather than trying to go cold turkey from the start, try replacing the extra, unnecessary calories with something like a hot cup of tea, a calorie-free Keto Snow Cone (page 256), or some Electrolyte Gummies (page 254). Or create a new habit like going for a nighttime stroll, taking a hot bath, or implementing a yoga or meditation routine.

Obsessing over the number on the scale. The scale can be a great tool for tracking progress, but it can also be discouraging for many people. If you're one of those people who steps on the scale three times a day and lets the number determine your mood for the next few hours, it's time to back away. Stop weighing yourself every single day and instead try once a week. The hour-to-hour and day-to-day variability of the number on the scale does not matter; it's the trend

QUIETING NEGATIVE THINKING

We're all human and we've all fallen into patterns of negative thinking. When making huge lifestyle changes like the one you are getting ready to make with the help of this book, it's only natural to get hung up on fears of failure or frustration that the scale isn't moving fast enough. But remember, the scale is not the be-all and end-all when it comes to weight loss and achieving optimal health. There are so many other factors, and being able to avoid and reverse negative thoughts or self-judgment is one of them.

If you constantly doubt your actions or shame yourself, you will have a hard time getting your mind on the same track as your goals. Finding ways to overcome negative feelings so they don't interfere with your progress is extremely important. Here are a few tips to get your mind right when those negative thoughts start taking over:

Acknowledge and move forward
When you start to feel yourself drifting toward a negative thought or feeling, don't just ignore it. Acknowledge why it's occurring and then shift your attention to something physical instead, like taking deep breaths, going for a walk, or texting or calling your friends or family to chat.

Analyze the thought logically
Rather than accepting the negative side, realize that there are probably some positives that you're failing to recognize. For example, is the number on the scale staying the same but your pants are feeling looser? Clearly something is happening there. Taking a more rational approach helps your brain see different perspectives.

Bump up the positivity every day
If you flood your brain with positive thoughts every day, it will be harder for the negative ones to take over. Every morning, write down three to five things you are grateful for. This will create a positive foundation to build the rest of your day upon.

over time that shows the real progress. Heck, sometimes I weigh myself, go to the bathroom, and weigh myself again and I've lost two pounds. Seriously, stop obsessing; it just messes with your head.

Letting the clock determine when you eat. Just because the clock hits noon doesn't mean you *have* to eat lunch. Are you actually hungry? Or are you just eating because you've trained your body to eat at the same time every day or because your coworkers are eating? At my old job, we had a strict lunch break from 12 to 12:45. As I became keto-adapted, I found myself not getting hungry until around 2 p.m. So instead of eating when I wasn't truly hungry, I filled that time period with a lunchtime walk while listening to a podcast. I then ate lunch at my desk later on in the afternoon when my body told me it was time.

Habits evolve over time, and being aware of them while also working toward replacing bad habits with new and better ones is what will determine how successful you'll be in the long run. This 21-day keto challenge includes a Weekly Wellness Tracker (page 84) to help you identify behaviors and patterns that may be helping or hindering your progress.

STAY MOTIVATED

We all know that it's easy to get excited and motivated at the onset of any commitment. But as we move forward, the excitement tends to dwindle and staying motivated becomes a little bit harder each day. This is completely normal and everyone goes through it, trust me. Here are a few tips and strategies for staying motivated:

Remember your why. You should establish your "why" from the start and remind yourself of it every day. Why are you embarking on this journey? Rather than just saying "to lose weight," figure out *why* you want or need to lose weight. Dig deeper and find the "why" that keeps you motivated no matter what.

Write down your goals and keep them in sight. Physically take pen to paper and write down your short- and long-term goals. Post them on your mirror so every day you see exactly what you're working toward.

Find a support group. You don't have to do this alone. There are thousands of people out there who are embarking on the same journey as you are right now! Seek out a friend or join an online community with people who have similar interests and goals as you. Check out my website (www.killinitketo.com) for more information on where to join keto support groups.

Establish a reward system . . . that isn't food! Positive reinforcement helps strengthen desirable behaviors. Give yourself small rewards as you reach those short-term goals. Stay away from rewards that involve food and instead choose rewards such as a relaxing pedicure or massage, a shopping spree, or a week-end getaway.

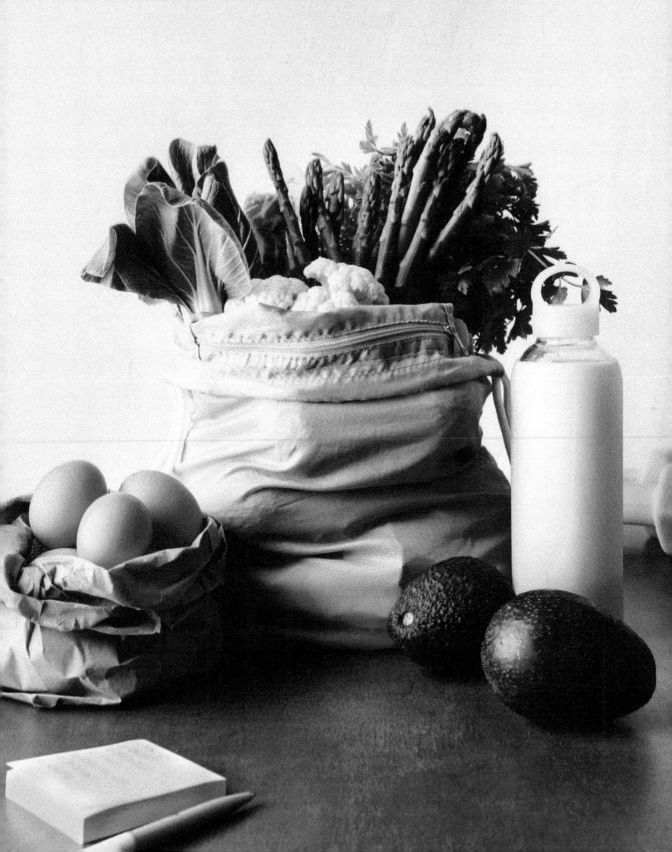

4

The 21-Day Challenge and Beyond

Now that you're familiar with what a ketogenic lifestyle entails and have reviewed the primary pillars of this challenge, it's finally time to get started! In this chapter, I provide you with several tools to guide you on your journey and help you form new, healthier habits. They say it takes 21 days to form a habit, so let's do this!

To make it as easy as possible for you, I've written up shopping lists and sample meal plans for each week, as well as tips and tricks to help you prep for the week ahead. The meal plans incorporate bulk recipes, so you'll have leftovers for quick weekday meals. Additional tools, like a Weekly Wellness Tracker, will help.

Remember, this 21-day program is designed to set you up for long-term success. It's not a quick-fix weight-loss plan. If you follow the guidelines, you will lose weight, but only by creating a healthier lifestyle will you be able to maintain that weight loss.

▶ Before You Begin

I know you're excited to get going, but before you begin your 21-day challenge, there are a few steps you need to take in order to set yourself up for success.

CLEAN OUT YOUR PANTRY

One of the biggest contributors to failure when starting any diet is having tempting and unhealthy foods around the house. The first step is to get rid of any foods or beverages that are not part of the plan. This will help eliminate triggers that may tempt you or interfere with your goals.

If you live with others who are not embarking on this journey with you, tell them that you are serious about this lifestyle change and that their support matters to you. Ask them to keep any non-keto-friendly foods in a separate cabinet or at least as far out of your sight as possible.

Foods to get rid of

Grains and starches: Bread, pasta, rice, oats, flour, cereal, corn, quinoa, bagels, wraps, cookies, crackers, potatoes, yams.

Beans and legumes: All beans, lentils, peas, chickpeas. Beans and legumes may provide nutrients, but aren't fit for a keto diet due to their high carb content.

Most fruit: Apples, bananas, pineapples, oranges, grapes, mangos, all fruit juices, dried fruits such as dates and raisins, fruit syrups, fruit concentrates, fruit smoothies.

Sugary foods and beverages: Honey, agave nectar, maple syrup, raw sugar, brown sugar, turbinado sugar, cane sugar, high fructose corn syrup, and anything that contains these sugars like desserts, pastries, candy, ice cream, milk chocolate, soda, etc.

Milk and low-fat dairy: Get rid of all milk, even whole milk, which few people realize contains 12 grams of sugar per cup. Toss any low-fat or fat-free cheeses, yogurts, or butter substitutes, and avoid pre-shredded cheeses that often contain potato starch.

Unhealthy fats and oils: Get rid of inflammatory and processed vegetable and seed oils including canola, corn, grapeseed, sunflower, safflower, and soybean oil and any items that include these, such as mayonnaise and salad dressings. Also toss out anything that is "hydrogenated" or "partially hydrogenated" like margarine and shortening.

Alcohol: I advise avoiding any alcohol throughout this challenge as it can slow down weight-loss efforts. But once you have completed the challenge and are adopting keto as a lifestyle, you can enjoy a glass of wine or a sugar-free cocktail as you please. Avoid higher carb alcohol like beer, sweet wines, flavored liquors, and sugary cocktails and mixers.

GO SHOPPING

Now that you've gotten rid of all the foods and beverages that are not on the plan, it's time to restock your pantry, refrigerator, and freezer with lots of keto-friendly options to help you crush this challenge and become the healthiest and happiest you've ever been.

There is a shopping list for each week of the challenge to help plan the recipes and meals for that week. In general, you'll want to stock up on the foods and beverages from the Complete Keto Foods List (page 25). The quantities provided in the weekly shopping lists are matched with the meal plan for that week for one person. If you are cooking for a family, be sure to adjust the ingredient quantities to fit your family's needs. To save time and money, I recommend buying your meats, seafood, eggs, frozen veggies, cheeses, and other pantry staples in bulk from stores like Costco or Sam's Club.

I also encourage you to read through the Keto-Specific Staples (page 28). There are some ingredients in the recipes that may seem foreign to you, but they can easily be purchased online or in many grocery stores.

PREP THE ESSENTIALS

There are some items that I advise prepping ahead of time before you start the challenge so they are ready to go for the entire 21-day period.

Spice blends: I recommend getting all of the ingredients together to make the "In a Hurry" Spice Blends (page 236). Making these spice blends ahead of time will make cooking so much easier and faster throughout the challenge. If you're cooking for a family, feel free to double or triple the spice blend recipes and store in large glass containers so you don't have to worry about running out.

Bone broth: Bone broth is used in many of the recipes because it is a great source of nutrients and adds tons of flavor to different dishes. I recommend making a batch or two of Bone Broth (page 240) and freezing it in 2- to 4-cup servings so you always have some on hand. If you're not interested in making your own, you can always buy high-quality bone broth online or in health food stores. I recommend the Kettle & Fire brand. The "broth" or "stock" that you find in your traditional grocery store is not actually made from real bones and is missing many of the nutrients and the flavor of *real* bone broth.

Browse the rest of the Staples chapter (page 235) for more prep-ahead options.

HOW TO USE THE MEAL PLANS

The meal plans provided for this challenge are meant to be used as a guide to help you establish a solid foundation for meal prepping and consuming the right types of food. By no means do you have to follow the meal plans exactly, and because all of the recipes provided are very low in total carbs, you can mix and match recipes as you see fit. Most of the recipes are also freezer-friendly, which is helpful when prepping for the weeks ahead.

The sample meal plans provide variation for those who need it, but for some, eating the same meals for breakfast, lunch, and dinner is more realistic and can be beneficial. If you are the type of person who does not need variety, I recommend choosing some of the bulk recipes and prepping them on a Sunday to enjoy for the entire week.

Additionally, the meal plans are not meant to be a one-size-fits-all eating plan. We are all individuals with different caloric needs and that is why I've designed the plans to leave room for adjusting serving sizes and incorporating suggested snacks when appropriate. Refer to the individual recipes for complete nutritional information and serving size suggestions.

If you plan on tracking your macros throughout the challenge, refer to page 16 for how to establish an appropriate starting calorie intake level and macronutrient distribution. Then, adjust the serving sizes for the recipes you choose to fit within your specific macro goals, and use the suggested snacks to fill in the gaps. If you do not plan on tracking macros, just make sure you are aware of your total daily carbohydrate intake (staying under 30 grams per day is a good place to start) and try your best to eat to satiety.

You'll also notice that I've included coffee in the breakfast section of each meal plan. This is because many people enjoy their morning coffee but tend to put the wrong things in it. Skip the sugar and skim milk and either enjoy it black or with a small amount of healthy fat, like heavy cream, MCT oil or powder, or coconut oil, as suggested. Feel free to swap the coffee for tea or leave it out altogether.

▶ Important Notes About the Recipes

In this book are over 100 easy and delicious recipes that are very low in total carbs (a vast majority are under 10 grams per serving) and completely compliant with a ketogenic lifestyle.

More than half of the recipes are Paleo or dairy-free or include options for making them Paleo or dairy-free.

We have included a number of recipe labels to help you navigate the recipe chapters and find the best recipes for you.

TIMING LABELS

Bulk Prep: These recipes make 6 to 12 servings and are freezable. Make these recipes when you want to stock your kitchen with delicious, ketogenic meals ready for the weeks and months ahead.

Under 30 Minutes: These recipes can be made in 30 minutes or less (including prep and cooking time).

DIETARY LABELS

Egg-Free   **Nut-Free**   **Paleo/Dairy-Free**   **Vegan**   **Vegetarian**

TIP LABELS

Recipes may include the following tips:

Recipe Tip: This tip offers general advice for the specific recipe.

Ingredient Tip: This tip offers advice for using specific ingredients and recommended brands.

Variation Tip: This tip offers advice for changing up the recipe. Change the protein, change the produce based on seasonality, change herbs for a different flavor profile, etc.

Make It Paleo/Dairy-Free: This tip offers advice for substituting or removing cheese and other dairy products to make the dish Paleo/Dairy-Free.

NUTRITION INFORMATION

You will find the nutritional information and macro breakdown **(in grams)** for each recipe. **The reason I do not recommend focusing on macro percentages is because they can be misleading and do not take into account quantity (calories).** Please be aware that the nutritional information may vary depending on the brands you are using. Make sure to also take into account any substitutions as well as serving size alterations when using this information.

Healthy cooking fats: Most of the recipes call for butter, ghee, or coconut oil to use when sautéing, but feel free to substitute any other stable cooking fat of your choice. See below for a guide to cooking with fats. Always choose organic, pastured, grass-fed and -finished when possible.

Best for medium to high heat

- Bacon fat
- Beef tallow
- Butter
- Coconut oil
- Ghee
- Lard

Best for salad dressings or very low heat

- Avocado oil
- Macadamia nut oil
- Olive oil
- Sesame oil

▶ Week 1

"A comfort zone is the most dangerous area anyone can stay in.
It is a place of no growth and no challenges."

—Brian Cagneey

The first week of keto is usually the hardest for most people because of the carbohydrate withdrawal. It will require you to step out of your comfort zone a bit. Some people experience symptoms of the "keto flu," such as headaches, fatigue, cravings, mood swings, and/or decreases in energy levels, but don't let this discourage you! Some people breeze through the first few days with no symptoms and others take a few days to get past them. The best way to ensure you get through the carb withdrawal phase without too much trouble is to make sure you stay hydrated, replenish your electrolytes (see page 42), consume enough healthy fats, and most importantly, *do not turn back to carbs* to try to relieve the symptoms.

If you follow these recommendations while sticking to the approved keto foods (page 25) and preparing for your first week in advance, you'll be on your way to ketosis and getting into that optimal fat-burning zone.

EXERCISE WEEK 1

If you're accustomed to a particular exercise routine, you may need to tone it down this week as your body adjusts to getting into ketosis. If you haven't exercised in a while, don't try to introduce a completely new routine this week. Stick with an easy walk during lunch or a light yoga session.

MEAL PREP

Taking a few hours on Sunday to prepare your meals for the week really helps with sticking to the plan. If you're cooking for one, freeze leftover portions for another week, or if you're cooking for a family, adjust the shopping list to fit your needs.

(Continued on page 86)

Step #1: Set 3 Goals for the next 21 days using the SMART goal template (page 69)

GOAL #1	GOAL #2	GOAL #3
S:	S:	S:
M:	M:	M:
A:	A:	A:
R:	R:	R:
T:	T:	T:

Step #2: Weight and Measurement Chart

The scale is a useful tool to show long-term progress but it doesn't give you the entire picture. Body measurements are a quick and easy way to see actual body composition changes as you progress through your journey. Record your starting weight and body measurements before you begin and then compare after you have completed the challenge.

Body Weight: Measure weight under the same conditions each time (immediately upon waking, no clothes, using the same scale).

Day 1: _____ **Day 21:** _____

Measurements: Using a tape measure, record your measurements according to the directions listed for each area (standing position).

· **Chest:** Measure with breath exhaled across the nipple.

Day 1: _____ **Day 21:** _____

· **Waist:** Measure the narrowest part of your midsection, just above your navel.

Day 1: _____ **Day 21:** _____

· **Hips:** Measure across the widest part of your hips and rear.

Day 1: _____ **Day 21:** _____

· **Thigh:** Measure around the largest point of your upper thigh.

Day 1: _____ **Day 21:** _____

Step #3: Take Before Pictures

I always encourage my clients to take before pictures so they can visually see how their bodies are changing. I've never had a client regret taking a before picture but have had many regret *not* taking them. Don't make that mistake!

Take three full-body pictures, front, side, and rear—men wearing only shorts and women wearing a sports bra and shorts or bikini.

Weekly Wellness Tracker Template*

	MONDAY	TUESDAY	WEDNESDAY
SLEEP	7.5 hours Hard to fall asleep; woke up one time during the night		
MOOD	Good energy throughout the day; minimal stress		
FASTING BLOOD GLUCOSE (OPTIONAL)	80 mg/dL		
KETONES (OPTIONAL)	1.3 mmol/L		
FOOD **TOTAL CARBS**	**B:** 2 Egg Muffins + coffee w/ 2 tbsp. cream **L:** 1 cup Tuna Salad + ½ avocado **D:** 1 serving Beef Stroganoff + 2 cups cauliflower rice + 1 tbsp. butter **S:** 1 oz. macadamia nuts + 2 electrolyte gummies **Total Carbs:** 28g		
WATER INTAKE (ONE DROPLET = 8 OZ.)	●●●●● ●●●○○	○○○○○ ○○○○○	○○○○○ ○○○○○
ELECTROLYTE INTAKE	Added sea salt to water + 1 packet electrolyte powder at 11 a.m.		
EXERCISE	· 20-minute walk during lunch · 45-minute evening yoga class		
HABIT	Replaced nighttime snack with a cup of hot tea		

*HOW TO USE YOUR WEEKLY WELLNESS TRACKER

Sleep: How many hours did you sleep? Did you have trouble falling asleep? Did you wake up feeling rested?

Mood: How was your overall mood today? Did you feel stressed? Did you have good energy throughout the day?

Fasting Blood Glucose (optional): If you are tracking your fasting blood glucose levels, note your reading each morning.

Ketones (optional): If you are tracking your ketone levels (see page 42), test at the same time each day and record your levels.

Food: Write down the food you ate for the day and include your total carbohydrate intake.

Water Intake: Check off how many glasses of water you drank throughout the day (1 water droplet = 8 ounces).

Electrolyte Intake: Note your electrolyte intake, whether that includes adding salt to your water or food or taking an electrolyte supplement. See page 40 for more details.

Exercise: Write down any physical activity or workouts you did during the day.

Habit: Write down one bad habit you replaced *or* a new habit you formed. You do not need to create a new habit every day. The idea is to work consistently at replacing a bad habit with a good one.

One of the perks to following a low-carbohydrate keto protocol is the decrease in hunger and reduction in cravings that make it ideal for losing weight. However, those who are more metabolically damaged or deal with dysregulated hunger hormones may benefit from implementing some of the hunger hacks listed below. These hunger hacks are very low-calorie, high-volume options that are great for warding off cravings without adding a ton of extra calories. They can help during times when willpower isn't enough.

- Keto Snow Cone (page 256)
- Electrolyte Gummies or jiggly flavored gelatin (page 254)
- Keto "Rice" Pudding (page 253)
- Mini Fat Bombs (page 247)
- Frozen Keto Coffee (page 117)
- Hot coffee or tea with 1 to 2 tablespoons healthy fats
- Sugar-free flavored sparkling water
- Stevia-sweetened soda (Zevia)
- Add 2 to 3 cups spinach or romaine lettuce to any meal

(Continued from page 81)

Follow these steps for prepping your first week's meals:

- Prepare the Cheesy Bacon Grab-and-Go Egg Muffins (page 126) and store the portion you will consume this week in an airtight container in the refrigerator. Freeze the remaining for another week.

- Make the Buffalo chicken for the Buffalo Chicken Salad (page 149) and prep the salad ingredients in containers or jars so they're ready to go for lunch.

- Prepare the Tuna Egg Salad (page 162) and portion out into small containers ready to go for lunch.

- Make the Beef Stroganoff (page 210).

- Prepare a batch of cauliflower rice for the week.

- Prep the snacks you'll be having this week and make sure to portion out recommended serving sizes.

WEEK 1 SHOPPING LIST

Meat and Seafood

- Bacon, 1 pound
- Beef sirloin, 1½ pounds
- Chicken thighs, boneless, skinless, 2 pounds
- Mahi mahi, 1 pound
- Tuna, packed in water, 2 (5-ounce) cans
- _____
- _____
- _____
- _____

Dairy, Dairy Alternatives, and Eggs

- Blue cheese or feta, 6 ounces
- Cheddar cheese, sharp, 4 ounces
- Coconut milk (unsweetened, full-fat, from a can), ½ cup
- Cream, heavy (whipping), 1 pint
- Eggs, large, 18
- Nut/seed milk (unsweetened hemp, almond, coconut, or cashew), ½ cup
- Parmesan cheese, 2 ounces
- Sour cream, ½ cup
- _____
- _____
- _____
- _____

Produce

- Avocados, 2
- Boston Bibb lettuce, 1 large head
- Broccoli florets, 4 cups (about 10 ounces)
- Cauliflower rice, fresh or frozen, 3 to 6 cups
- Garlic, 3 cloves
- Lemon, 1
- Mushrooms, 8 ounces
- Onion, 1 small
- Parsley, fresh, 1 bunch
- Romaine lettuce, 12 cups
- Spinach, 1 cup
- _____
- _____
- _____
- _____
- _____
- _____

Pantry, Refrigerator, Freezer Staples

- Almond flour or crushed pork rinds
- Bone Broth (page 240)
- Butter or ghee
- Cacao/cocoa powder, unsweetened
- Cayenne pepper
- Coconut oil or lard (or other cooking fat, see page 27)
- Coffee or tea
- Dijon mustard
- Everything Seasoning (page 236) or store-bought
- Garlic powder
- Harissa paste
- Hot sauce
- Macadamia nuts
- Mayonnaise
- MCT powder or oil
- Onion powder
- Oregano, dried
- Pepper, black
- Pepper, red flakes
- Ranch dressing
- Sea salt
- Sunflower seeds, hulled
- Sweetener
- Xanthan gum or guar gum
- _____
- _____
- _____
- _____
- _____
- _____
- _____
- _____
- _____
- _____
- _____
- _____
- _____

Snack Suggestions

Week 1 Snacks

Choose two or three snacks from the list below and check your refrigerator/freezer/pantry for items or add them to your grocery list.

- Cheese cubes (1 ounce per serving)
- Cheese crisps
- Electrolyte Gummies (page 254)

- Hard-boiled eggs (1 or 2 per serving)
- Macadamia nuts (1 ounce per serving)
- Mini Fat Bombs (page 247)

- Olives (7 to 9 large olives per serving)
- Pork rinds
- _____
- _____

Week 2 Snacks

Choose one or two snacks from the list below and check your refrigerator/freezer/pantry for items or add them to your grocery list. You can also choose snacks from week 1.

- almonds (23 per serving) or other low-carb nuts or seeds
- Dill Deviled Eggs (page 139)
- Easy Cheesy Sausage Balls (page 130)
- Keto Snow Cone (page 256)

- Quick Keto Blender Muffins (page 120)
- salami (1 ounce per serving)
- _____
- _____
- _____

- _____
- _____
- _____
- _____
- _____

Week 3 Snacks

Try to limit the snacking this week to just one per day. Choose one snack from the list below and check your refrigerator/freezer/pantry for items or add them to your grocery list. You can also choose snacks from weeks 1 and 2.

- Keto Antipasto (page 141)
- Loaded Bacon and Cheddar Cheese Balls (page 145)
- Pili nuts (1 ounce per serving)
- Bone Broth (page 240)
- _____

- _____
- _____
- _____
- _____
- _____

- _____
- _____
- _____
- _____
- _____

Week 1 Meal Plan

	BREAKFAST	LUNCH	DINNER
MONDAY	Cheesy Bacon Grab-and-Go Egg Muffins (page 126) Coffee with 1 to 2 tablespoons heavy cream or MCT oil/powder	Buffalo Chicken Salad (page 149)	Beef Stroganoff (page 210) over 1 to 2 cups cauliflower rice sautéed in 1 tablespoon butter or ghee
TUESDAY	Cheesy Bacon Grab-and-Go Egg Muffins Coffee with 1 to 2 tablespoons heavy cream or MCT oil/powder	Tuna Egg Salad (page 162) served in half a medium avocado (about 75 grams)	Harissa Coconut Chicken (page 177) in 4 large Boston Bibb lettuce leaves
WEDNESDAY	Keto Flu Combat Smoothie (page 114) Coffee with 1 to 2 tablespoons heavy cream	Buffalo Chicken Salad	Beef Stroganoff over 1 to 2 cups cauliflower rice sautéed in 1 tablespoon butter or ghee
THURSDAY	Cheesy Bacon Grab-and-Go Egg Muffins Coffee with 1 to 2 tablespoons heavy cream or MCT oil/powder	Tuna Egg Salad served in half medium avocado (about 75 grams)	Harissa Coconut Chicken over 1 to 2 cups cauliflower rice sautéed in 1 tablespoon butter or ghee
FRIDAY	Keto Flu Combat Smoothie Coffee with 1 to 2 tablespoons heavy cream	Buffalo Chicken Salad	Beef Stroganoff Zesty Roasted Broccoli (page 227)
SATURDAY	BAE Breakfast Bowl (page 129) Coffee with 1 to 2 tablespoons heavy cream or MCT oil/powder	Tuna Egg Salad 1 serving Zesty Roasted Broccoli	Simple Nut-Crusted Mahi Mahi (page 163) served with side salad using chopped Boston Bibb + 1 to 2 tablespoons ranch
SUNDAY	Skip and enjoy lunch as "brunch" Coffee with 1 to 2 tablespoons heavy cream plus 1 tablespoon MCT oil/powder or coconut oil	BAE Breakfast Bowl	Simple Nut-Crusted Mahi Mahi Zesty Roasted Broccoli Or meal from Week 2 Meal Prep

Guidelines for Water and Electrolyte Consumption: Consume **at least** 8 (8-ounce) glasses of water per day. Add sea salt to your water and food (this is very important, especially during the first week to combat keto flu symptoms). Follow the guidelines on page 41.

Weekly Wellness Tracker

	MONDAY	TUESDAY	WEDNESDAY
SLEEP			
MOOD			
FASTING BLOOD GLUCOSE (OPTIONAL)			
KETONES (OPTIONAL)			
FOOD			
TOTAL CARBS			
WATER INTAKE (ONE DROPLET = 8 OZ.)	○ ○ ○ ○ ○ ○ ○ ○ ○ ○	○ ○ ○ ○ ○ ○ ○ ○ ○ ○	○ ○ ○ ○ ○ ○ ○ ○ ○ ○
ELECTROLYTE INTAKE			
EXERCISE			
HABIT			

THURSDAY	FRIDAY	SATURDAY	SUNDAY
◊ ◊ ◊ ◊ ◊ ◊ ◊ ◊ ◊ ◊	◊ ◊ ◊ ◊ ◊ ◊ ◊ ◊ ◊ ◊	◊ ◊ ◊ ◊ ◊ ◊ ◊ ◊ ◊ ◊	◊ ◊ ◊ ◊ ◊ ◊ ◊ ◊ ◊ ◊

▶ Week 2

"Success is the sum of small efforts, repeated day in and day out."

—Robert Collier

Congratulations on making it through week 1! Now that the carb withdrawal phase is out of the way, things should start to get a bit easier each day and you should begin to feel some of the amazing effects of being in a state of ketosis—better mood, stable energy levels, appetite suppression, and more.

The focus for week 2 is staying consistent. You're now familiar with the foods you should be consuming and those that need to be avoided. Take some time to reflect on week 1: Look back at your Weekly Wellness Tracker and review your goals. Think about what you can do differently this week to make things easier while still sticking to the plan. Did you prep enough food? Did you replenish your electrolytes? Use what you learned from week 1 to ensure week 2 goes even more smoothly.

EXERCISE WEEK 2

If you're accustomed to a usual workout routine, start to introduce it back into your daily activity. If you're just getting into a routine, try to follow it at least three days this week. Use the recommended exercises on page 55 as a guide to start incorporating more strength and cardiovascular movements into your weekly workout plan. Make sure you are still replenishing your electrolytes this week and staying hydrated, especially surrounding physical activities.

MEAL PREP

If you have leftovers from last week that you enjoyed and would like to eat this week, make sure to defrost them ahead of time. Go through this week's menu and plan your meals for breakfast, lunch, dinner, and snacks (if needed).

Here are some guidelines for prepping week 2 meals:

- Make the Slow Cooker Pulled Pork (page 194).

- Prepare the Sausage, Spinach, and Goat Cheese Breakfast Casserole (page 128). Once cooled, cut into squares and store this week's portion in an airtight container in the refrigerator and freeze the remaining for another week.

- Make the Greek Salad in a Jar (page 150), following the directions for assembly and storing in the refrigerator for a quick grab-and-go lunch.

- Make the Asian Fusion Sauce (page 195) to go with the pulled pork.

- If making Chesos (page 200), decide which toppings you'd like to use and add them to your grocery list.

- If making the Overnight "Noats" (page 116), make sure you have all the ingredients on hand and decide which toppings you'd like to add.

- Prep the snacks you'll be having for the week and make sure to portion out recommended serving sizes.

WEEK 2 SHOPPING LIST

Meat and Seafood

- Bacon, 8 slices
- Beef sirloin or flank, 1 pound
- Breakfast sausage or ground pork, 1 pound
- Pork rinds, 2 cups
- Pork shoulder, 1 (4- to 6-pound) boneless

Dairy, Dairy Alternatives, and Eggs

- Cheddar cheese, 10 ounces
- Cream, heavy (whipping), 1 pint
- Cream cheese, 16 ounces
- Eggs, large, 20
- Feta cheese, 4 ounces
- Goat cheese, 5 ounces
- Nut/seed milk, unsweetened (hemp, almond, coconut, cashew), 1 cup
- Sour cream, 1 tablespoon

Produce

- Baby bok choy, 24 ounces (about 12 small heads)
- Broccoli florets, 2 cups
- Cherry tomatoes, 8
- Cucumbers, 2
- Garlic, 2 heads
- Olives, 16
- Onion (large), 1
- Romaine lettuce, 4 cups
- Spinach, frozen, 1 (10-ounce) package

Pantry, Refrigerator, Freezer Staples (Check On-Hand Supplies)

- Baking powder
- Bone Broth (page 240)
- Butter or ghee
- Cayenne pepper
- Chia seeds
- Chili paste
- Chili powder
- Cinnamon, ground
- Coconut aminos
- Coconut flour
- Coconut oil or lard
- Coconut vinegar or apple Cider vinegar
- Coffee or tea
- Collagen powder
- Cumin, ground
- Dijon mustard, 2 teaspoons
- Fat-Burning Dressing (page 238)
- Fish sauce
- Garlic powder
- Ginger, ground
- Hemp seeds (hulled)
- "In a Hurry" Spice Blend of choice or fresh herbs
- Liquid aminos or tamari
- Mayonnaise
- Mexican Spice Blend (page 237)
- MCT oil
- MCT powder (optional if you already have oil)
- Nut butter or sugar-free syrup
- Nutmeg, ground
- Olives (large), 16
- Onion powder
- Pepper, black
- Pepper, red flakes
- Pickled jalapeños
- Pork rinds, 2 cups
- Salsa (optional)
- Sea salt
- Sesame oil
- Sesame seeds (optional)
- Sweetener
- Vanilla extract, pure
- Xanthan gum or guar gum

Snack Suggestions

See p. 88.

Week 2 Meal Plan

	BREAKFAST	LUNCH	DINNER
MONDAY	Sausage, Spinach, and Goat Cheese Breakfast Casserole (page 128) Coffee with 1 to 2 tablespoons heavy cream or MCT oil/powder	Greek Salad in a Jar (page 150)	Slow Cooker Pulled Pork with Asian Fusion Sauce (page 194) Garlic Butter Baby Bok Choy (page 226)
TUESDAY	Overnight "Noats" (page 116) Coffee with 1 to 2 tablespoons heavy cream or MCT oil/powder	Greek Salad in a Jar	Chesos (Cheese Shell Tacos) Carnitas (page 200)
WEDNESDAY	Skip and enjoy breakfast for lunch Coffee with 1 to 2 tablespoons heavy cream plus 1 tablespoon MCT oil/powder or coconut oil	Sausage, Spinach, and Goat Cheese Breakfast Casserole	Slow Cooker Pulled Pork with Asian Fusion Sauce Garlic Butter Baby Bok Choy
THURSDAY	Overnight "Noats" Coffee with 1 to 2 tablespoons heavy cream or MCT oil/powder	Greek Salad in a Jar	Chesos (Cheese Shell Tacos) Carnitas
FRIDAY	Sausage, Spinach, and Goat Cheese Breakfast Casserole Coffee with 1 to 2 tablespoons heavy cream or MCT oil/powder	Greek Salad in a Jar	Better than Take-Out Beef with Broccoli (page 204)
SATURDAY	Skip and enjoy lunch as "brunch" Coffee with 2 tablespoons heavy cream plus 1 tablespoon coconut oil or MCT oil/powder	Easy Skillet Pancakes (page 119) or Quick Keto Blender Muffins (page 120) 1 to 2 tablespoons nut butter or sugar-free syrup	Pork Rind Nachos (page 193) made with leftover carnitas
SUNDAY	Skip and enjoy lunch as "brunch" Coffee with 2 tablespoons heavy cream plus 1 tablespoon coconut oil or MCT oil/powder	Easy Skillet Pancakes 1 to 2 tablespoons nut butter or sugar-free syrup	Better than Take-Out Beef with Broccoli Or Meal from Week 3 Meal Prep

Guidelines for Water and Electrolyte Consumption: Consume **at least** 8 (8-ounce) glasses of water per day. Add sea salt to your water and food. Follow the guidelines on page 41.

Weekly Wellness Tracker

	MONDAY	TUESDAY	WEDNESDAY
SLEEP			
MOOD			
FASTING BLOOD GLUCOSE (OPTIONAL)			
KETONES (OPTIONAL)			
FOOD			
TOTAL CARBS			
WATER INTAKE (ONE DROPLET = 8 OZ.)	○ ○ ○ ○ ○ ○ ○ ○ ○ ○	○ ○ ○ ○ ○ ○ ○ ○ ○ ○	○ ○ ○ ○ ○ ○ ○ ○ ○ ○
ELECTROLYTE INTAKE			
EXERCISE			
HABIT			

THURSDAY	FRIDAY	SATURDAY	SUNDAY
◊ ◊ ◊ ◊ ◊ ◊ ◊ ◊ ◊ ◊	◊ ◊ ◊ ◊ ◊ ◊ ◊ ◊ ◊ ◊	◊ ◊ ◊ ◊ ◊ ◊ ◊ ◊ ◊ ◊	◊ ◊ ◊ ◊ ◊ ◊ ◊ ◊ ◊ ◊

▶ Week 3

The last week of your 21-day challenge is here! By now you should be feeling pretty great and embracing the increased energy and mental clarity. You should also have fewer cravings for sugary foods and processed carbs. As you dive into week 3, think about how far you have already come in just a short period of time. Reflect on your Weekly Wellness Trackers and all that you've learned so far on your journey. What improvements can you make this week to help you further progress toward your goals?

Now that you've started to tap into your body fat stores for energy, try experimenting with intermittent fasting (page 35) a few days this week. Focus on becoming more aware of your true hunger signals and start to find an eating schedule that works for your personal lifestyle.

EXERCISE WEEK 3

Energy levels should be high this week, which means getting in a bit more physical activity won't be too difficult. Try to push yourself a little bit more during your workouts and begin to establish a routine that is both enjoyable and challenging. If you're following the recommended exercise routines from page 55, try adding a few more reps or increase the weight slightly from last week. Keep up the recommended hydration and electrolyte intake.

MEAL PREP

By now you should be finding recipes and combinations of foods that you enjoy and find satisfying. Make the most of leftovers or try out some of the new recipes from this week's meal plan.

Here are some guidelines for prepping week 3 meals:

- Make the Quick Keto Blender Muffins (page 120) and store in the refrigerator.

- Prepare the Jalapeño Bacon Egg Salad (page 151).

- Prep the ingredients for making a half recipe of the Special Sauce Cobb Salad (page 148).

- Make sure the Indian Spice Blend (page 236) is made and prep the chicken for the Quick Keto Butter Chicken (page 183).

- Prepare a batch of cauliflower rice for the week or swap for a different non-starchy vegetable.

- Prep the snacks you'll be having for the week (if needed) and make sure to portion out recommended serving sizes.

WEEK 3 SHOPPING LIST

Meat and Seafood

- Bacon, 14 slices
- Breakfast sausage or ground pork, 12 ounces
- Chicken, rotisserie, 1
- Chicken thighs, boneless, skinless, 1 pound
- Chorizo, loose, 1 pound
- Ground beef, 2 pounds
- Ground pork, 1 pound
- _____
- _____
- _____
- _____

Dairy, Dairy Alternatives, and Eggs

- Cheddar cheese, sharp, 10 ounces
- Cream cheese, 12 ounces
- Cream, heavy (whipping), 1 pint
- Eggs, large, 19
- Mozzarella cheese, 6 ounces
- Sour cream, 1 cup
- _____
- _____
- _____

Produce

- Avocados, 2
- Boston Bibb lettuce, 1 head
- Cauliflower rice, fresh or frozen, 4 cups
- Cherry tomatoes, 4
- Chives, fresh, 1 bunch
- Garlic, 4 cloves
- Green chile peppers, 2 (or 1 [4-ounce] can)
- Jalapeño pepper, 1
- Lime, 1
- Onions, 2
- Romaine lettuce or spinach, 4 cups
- _____
- _____
- _____
- _____
- _____

Pantry, Refrigerator, Freezer Staples

- Almond flour
- Baking powder
- Bone Broth (page 240)
- Butter or ghee
- Chili powder
- Cinnamon, ground
- Coconut flour
- Coconut oil or lard
- Coconut vinegar or apple cider vinegar
- Coffee or tea
- Collagen powder
- Cumin, ground
- Everything Seasoning (page 236) or store-bought
- Garam masala
- Garlic powder
- Gelatin or xanthan gum or guar gum
- Ginger, ground
- Hot sauce
- Mayonnaise
- MCT powder or oil
- Mexican Spice Blend
- Nut butter
- Nutmeg, ground
- Onion powder
- Paprika
- Pepper, black
- Pork rinds, 1 cup crushed (if using for Keto Dough)
- Sea salt
- Sweetener
- Tomato paste
- Turmeric, ground

Snack Suggestions

See p. 88.

Week 3 Meal Plan

	BREAKFAST	LUNCH	DINNER
MONDAY	"Fat Fast" until lunch: Frozen Keto Coffee (page 117) or coffee with 1 to 2 table-spoons heavy cream or MCT oil/powder	Jalapeño Bacon Egg Salad (page 151) served in half medium avocado (about 75 grams)	Quick Keto Butter Chicken (page 183) over 1 to 2 cups cauliflower rice sautéed in 1 tablespoon butter or ghee
TUESDAY	Quick Keto Blender Muffins (page 120) with 1 to 2 tablespoons nut butter	Special Sauce Cobb Salad (page 148)	Special Chorizo with Avocado Crema (page 206) served in lettuce cups
WEDNESDAY	"Fat Fast" until lunch: Frozen Keto Coffee or coffee with 1 to 2 tablespoons heavy cream or MCT oil/powder	Jalapeño Bacon Egg Salad served in half medium avocado (about 75 grams)	Quick Keto Butter Chicken over 1 to 2 cups cauliflower rice sautéed in 1 tablespoon butter or ghee
THURSDAY	Quick Keto Blender Muffins with 1 to 2 tablespoons nut butter	Special Sauce Cobb Salad	Special Chorizo with Avocado Crema served in lettuce cups
FRIDAY	"Fat Fast" until lunch: Frozen Keto Coffee or coffee with 1 to 2 tablespoons heavy cream or MCT oil/powder	Jalapeño Bacon Egg Salad served in lettuce cups	Buffalo Chicken Pizza (page 178) (use leftover chicken from week 1 or make fresh)
SATURDAY	Skip and enjoy lunch as "brunch" Coffee with 1 to 2 table-spoons heavy cream or MCT oil/powder	Keto Biscuits and Gravy (page 122) or leftover Buffalo Chicken Pizza	Meaty Keto Chili (page 157)
SUNDAY	Skip and enjoy lunch as "brunch" Coffee with 1 to 2 table-spoons heavy cream or MCT oil/powder	Keto Biscuits and Gravy	Meaty Keto Chili

Guidelines for Water and Electrolyte Consumption: Consume **at least** 8 (8-ounce) glasses of water per day. Add sea salt to your water and food. Follow the guidelines on page 41.

Weekly Wellness Tracker

	MONDAY	TUESDAY	WEDNESDAY
SLEEP			
MOOD			
FASTING BLOOD GLUCOSE (OPTIONAL)			
KETONES (OPTIONAL)			
FOOD			
TOTAL CARBS			
WATER INTAKE (ONE DROPLET = 8 OZ.)	○○○○○ ○○○○○	○○○○○ ○○○○○	○○○○○ ○○○○○
ELECTROLYTE INTAKE			
EXERCISE			
HABIT			

THURSDAY	FRIDAY	SATURDAY	SUNDAY
⬡ ⬡ ⬡ ⬡ ⬡ ⬡ ⬡ ⬡ ⬡ ⬡	⬡ ⬡ ⬡ ⬡ ⬡ ⬡ ⬡ ⬡ ⬡ ⬡	⬡ ⬡ ⬡ ⬡ ⬡ ⬡ ⬡ ⬡ ⬡ ⬡	⬡ ⬡ ⬡ ⬡ ⬡ ⬡ ⬡ ⬡ ⬡ ⬡

▶ Make It a Lifestyle

Congratulations! You made it through the 21-Day Keto Challenge! I hope you have had success over these past three weeks and learned how powerful this way of eating can truly be. The challenge is over, but it doesn't stop here.

Now that you've mastered the keto basics and taken control of the other areas of your health—exercise, sleep, stress management, and mind-set—you can begin to incorporate what you've learned into your everyday life. You committed to this challenge and completed it, and now it's time to commit to becoming the best version of yourself. Going forward, continue to embrace the strategies you implemented during the challenge—goal setting, planning, mindfulness, healthy eating, habit changes, and anything else you learned along the way. You'll soon realize that a low-carbohydrate lifestyle is the optimal way to live and it will become second nature for you.

ADJUSTING PRIORITIES

In the last 21 days you've made a choice to prioritize a healthy lifestyle. You worked hard at changing your eating style, replacing bad habits with good ones, and setting goals to maximize your health and wellness, both mentally and physically. Keeping up this shift in mind-set will help you continue to build on the progress that you've already made.

There are going to be bumps in the road and there may even be people who try to sabotage what you've worked hard for. The key to finding long-term success is to block out all the noise as best you can and continue to remind yourself why you started this journey. Be selfish, be strict, and pay close attention to what you need to do to achieve and maintain your goals.

Be stronger than your excuses.

We all make excuses to try to justify things that we didn't do or fell short of achieving. Don't allow yourself that luxury. Yes, making time to meal prep, tracking food, exercise, changing habits, and staying on track is not going to be a walk in the park. But every excuse you make will only set you back and derail you from achieving your best self. Leave the excuses behind and continue to prioritize your goals. Use the tools you've learned during this program to grow your healthy habits and strive for consistency rather than perfection. Remember, trust the process!

TIPS FOR LONG-TERM SUCCESS

It's not easy going "against the norm" and it's going to take a little bit of extra effort until your new lifestyle starts to feel second nature to you. But I promise, if you're consistent and continue to embrace all that you've learned from this challenge, you'll be on your way to crushing those long-term goals and maintaining a healthy and stable weight with improved overall health.

Here are a few tips for achieving long-term success with a low-carbohydrate, ketogenic lifestyle:

Focus on consistency, not perfection. Not every day is going to be perfect and that's just part of life. Long-term success comes from staying consistent each week and finding a routine that's sustainable but also enjoyable.

Don't restrict, replace. Stop thinking about the things you "can't" have and start finding replacements. This is a big part of making keto a lifestyle. Craving pizza? Make Buffalo Chicken Pizza (page 178) or Pizza Bagel Bites (page 137). Craving a brownie? Make some Fudgy Keto Brownies (page 260). This lifestyle is not restrictive—there is always an alternative. Check out the Keto Alternatives page on my website (www.killinitketo.com) for more ideas.

Join a support group. You aren't in this alone. There are tons of people out there who are embarking on the same journey as you, and connecting with them to share ideas, questions, and concerns is a great way to learn and stay on track. Consider joining my online challenge to be part of the virtual community that we've created to offer long-term support and guidance.

Ignore the haters. There are many people out there who do not understand the keto lifestyle and therefore try to justify why it's wrong or doesn't work. These people are either misinformed or may have an ulterior motive. Don't let what they say get to you or influence your ability to progress toward a healthier and happier you.

Stop using the word "diet." Diets are short term and often associated with restriction and negativity. Keto may have started off as a "diet" for you, but it's time to start shifting that mentality and adopting this way of eating as a lifestyle. If you do this, the benefits will continue to stack up and you'll realize why this lifestyle is so powerful for achieving long-term health and wellness.

Don't compare yourself to others. One of the biggest mistakes you can make is trying to replicate exactly what someone else is doing or falling into the one-size-fits-all mentality. We are all individuals and what works for one person may not work for another. You have to experiment and find ways to make this lifestyle work for you and your goals.

Celebrate your success. Look back at how far you have come. Not just with weight loss but with other areas of your life such as stress, sleep, habits, exercise, energy levels, and confidence, too. All of these things add up to creating a healthier and happier you. Share your success with others and continue to work toward your goals each day.

MAKE YOUR OWN WEEKLY MENU

Now that you're a keto pro and have found the foods and recipes that you enjoy most, I invite you to create your own personal weekly menu. Remember to keep in mind your total daily carb count and try to avoid excessive snacking throughout the day.

Meal Plan

	BREAKFAST	LUNCH	DINNER
MONDAY			
TUESDAY			
WEDNESDAY			
THURSDAY			
FRIDAY			
SATURDAY			
SUNDAY			

Weekly Wellness Tracker

	MONDAY	TUESDAY	WEDNESDAY
SLEEP			
MOOD			
FASTING BLOOD GLUCOSE (OPTIONAL)			
KETONES (OPTIONAL)			
FOOD			
TOTAL CARBS			
WATER INTAKE (ONE DROPLET = 8 OZ.)	○ ○ ○ ○ ○ ○ ○ ○ ○ ○	○ ○ ○ ○ ○ ○ ○ ○ ○ ○	○ ○ ○ ○ ○ ○ ○ ○ ○ ○
ELECTROLYTE INTAKE			
EXERCISE			
HABIT			

THURSDAY	FRIDAY	SATURDAY	SUNDAY
◊ ◊ ◊ ◊ ◊ ◊ ◊ ◊ ◊ ◊	◊ ◊ ◊ ◊ ◊ ◊ ◊ ◊ ◊ ◊	◊ ◊ ◊ ◊ ◊ ◊ ◊ ◊ ◊ ◊	◊ ◊ ◊ ◊ ◊ ◊ ◊ ◊ ◊ ◊

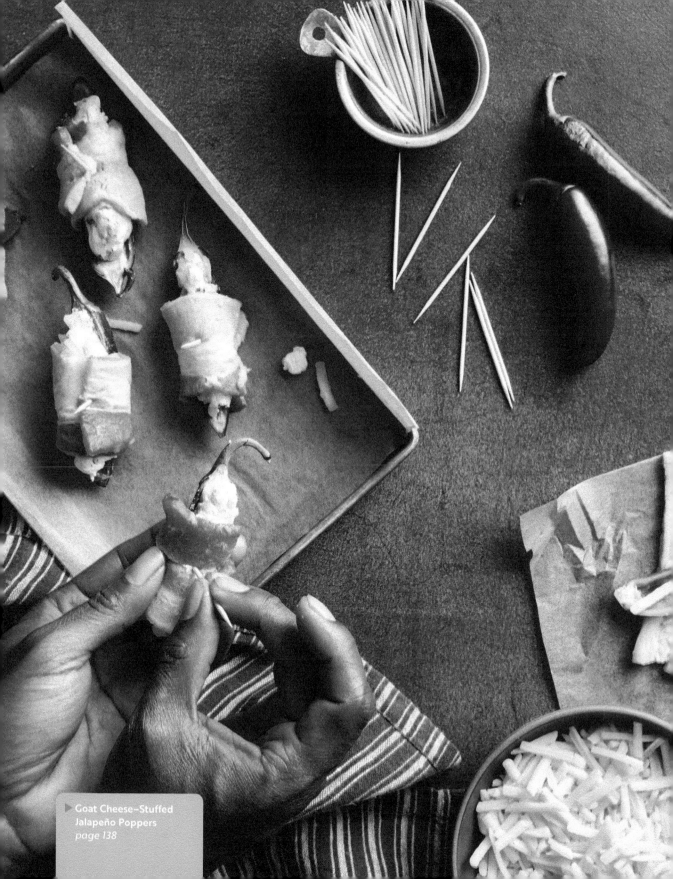

Goat Cheese–Stuffed
Jalapeño Poppers
page 138

PART TWO

The Recipes

THE HARDEST PART about any change in your diet, especially a change as significant as keto, is figuring out not only what you can and can't eat, but what you can eat that will give you joy and leave you feeling truly satisfied. The rest of this book is filled with recipes for delicious, satisfying, nutritious foods that will leave your belly full and your taste buds happy!

There are recipes here for every meal of the day, as well as for snacks, staples, and treats. While I encourage you to keep it simple during the first 21 days and limit keto treats, as you steadily adopt a keto lifestyle, you can begin to incorporate more tasty recipes from this book that will soon become favorites in your weekly meal planning. You'll find a variety of common dishes that have been "keto-fied," such as pancakes, bagels, tacos, pizza, and many more. I'm confident you'll soon realize that this way of eating is not restrictive and the possibilities for delicious, keto-friendly options are infinite!

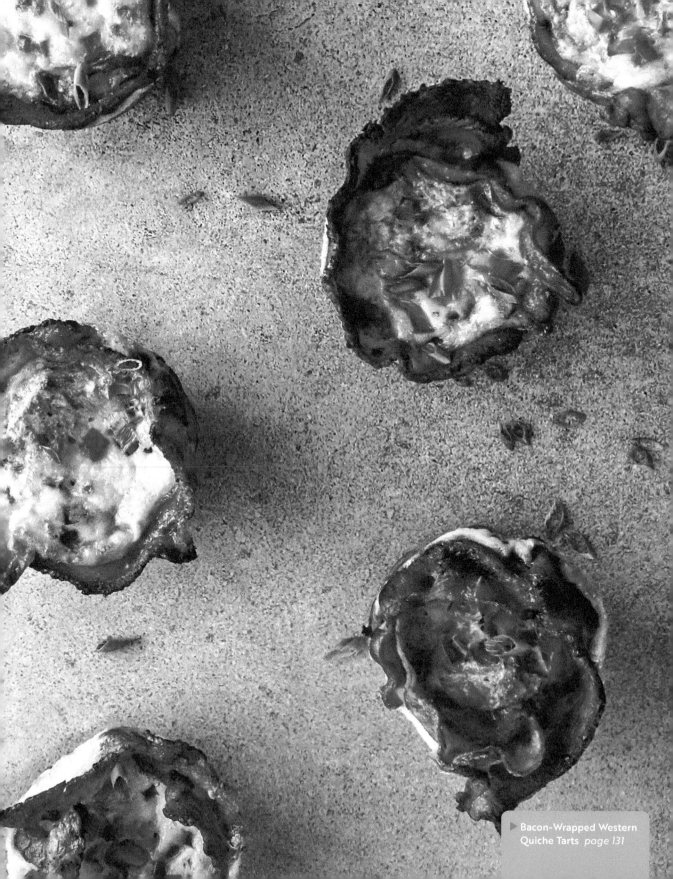

► Bacon-Wrapped Western
Quiche Tarts *page 131*

5

Smoothies and Breakfast

KETO FLU COMBAT SMOOTHIE

SERVES 1 | PREP TIME: 5 MINUTES

EGG-FREE · **NUT-FREE** · **PALEO/DAIRY-FREE** · **VEGAN** · **UNDER 30 MINUTES**

Need a quick and easy way to replenish those electrolytes? This smoothie is packed with the vital nutrients needed to combat that dreaded "keto flu" (see page 40). It's a tad higher in carbohydrates than many of the other recipes in this book, but that's due to the avocado. They have some carbs, but avocados are considered a superfood in the keto world, loaded with healthy fats, fiber, and several vitamins and minerals.

½ cup unsweetened nut or seed milk (hemp, almond, coconut, cashew)

1 cup spinach

½ medium avocado (about 75 grams), pitted and peeled

1 scoop MCT powder (or 1 tablespoon MCT oil)

½ tablespoon unsweetened cacao powder

¼ teaspoon sea salt

Dash sweetener (optional)

½ cup ice

In a blender, combine the milk, spinach, avocado, MCT powder, cacao powder, salt, sweetener (if using), and ice and blend until smooth.

INGREDIENT TIP: I like to use Perfect Keto chocolate- or vanilla-flavored MCT powder when making this smoothie.

PER SERVING

Calories: 249; Total Fat: 21g; Protein: 5g; Total Carbs: 10g; Fiber: 8g; Net Carbs: 2g

STRAWBERRIES AND CREAM SMOOTHIE

SERVES 1 | PREP TIME: 5 MINUTES

EGG-FREE · **NUT-FREE** · **VEGETARIAN** · **UNDER 30 MINUTES**

This smoothie is a sweet blend of antioxidant-rich strawberries and a blast of fats that will keep you ketogenic while satisfying your sweet tooth. This recipe works great first thing in the morning as a replacement for yogurt, or as an after-dinner treat.

5 medium strawberries, hulled

3 tablespoons heavy (whipping) cream

3 ice cubes

Your favorite vanilla-flavored sweetener

In a blender, combine all the ingredients and blend until smooth. Enjoy right **away!**

VARIATION TIP: If you don't have a vanilla-flavored sweetener, ⅛ teaspoon of vanilla extract will do the trick.

PER SERVING (1 shake)

Calories: 176; Total Fat: 16g; Protein: 2g; Total Carbs: 6g; Fiber: 1g; Net Carbs: 5g

OVERNIGHT "NOATS"

SERVES 1 | PREP TIME: 5 MINUTES PLUS OVERNIGHT TO CHILL

EGG-FREE · NUT-FREE · PALEO/DAIRY-FREE · VEGAN

Before keto, I used to make overnight oatmeal for breakfast during the week. It was easy, quick, and I could mix up the flavors in so many ways that I never got bored. Keto "noats" are perfect for replacing traditional oats and will keep you full and satisfied longer than those regular sugar-spiking oats would. Add different flavors like unsweetened cacao, cinnamon, vanilla extract, stevia, or monk fruit and top with chopped nuts, nut butter, or a few berries.

2 tablespoons hulled hemp seeds

1 tablespoon chia seeds

½ scoop (about 8 grams) collagen powder

½ cup unsweetened nut or seed milk (hemp, almond, coconut, cashew)

1. In a small mason jar or glass container, combine the hemp seeds, chia seeds, collagen, and milk.

2. Secure tightly with a lid, shake well, and refrigerate overnight.

INGREDIENT TIP: I use the Perfect Keto brand chocolate- or vanilla-flavored collagen powder for this recipe because it is mixed with MCT powder, yielding an ideal fat-to-protein ratio. If using other collagen powders, be aware that the protein and fat ratios will vary, and adjust accordingly.

BULK PREP TIP: Double, triple, or quadruple the ingredients and divide into small jars for easy grab-and-go breakfasts during the week.

PER SERVING

Calories: 263; Total Fat: 19g; Protein: 16g; Total Carbs: 7g; Fiber: 5g; Net Carbs: 2g

FROZEN KETO COFFEE

SERVES 1 | PREP TIME: 5 MINUTES

EGG-FREE · NUT-FREE · PALEO/DAIRY-FREE OPTION · UNDER 30 MINUTES

Did you know that one grande vanilla frappuccino from Starbucks has 69 grams of sugar and more than 400 calories? Not the best option to start your day, if you ask me. Try this frozen keto coffee instead. The combination of coffee and MCT powder will boost your energy and ketones while keeping you satisfied all morning long. It's also a great option for an afternoon pick-me-up.

12 ounces coffee, chilled

1 scoop MCT powder (or 1 tablespoon MCT oil)

1 tablespoon heavy (whipping) cream

Pinch ground cinnamon

Dash sweetener (optional)

½ cup ice

In a blender, combine the coffee, MCT powder, cream, cinnamon, sweetener (if using), and ice. Blend until smooth.

INGREDIENT TIP: I use Perfect Keto unflavored MCT powder for this frozen keto coffee but you can also use the flavored versions if you like.

MAKE IT PALEO/DAIRY-FREE: Substitute ghee or coconut milk/cream for the heavy cream.

PER SERVING

Calories: 127; Total Fat: 13g; Protein: 1g; Total Carbs: 1.5g; Fiber: 1g; Net Carbs: 0.5g

NO-BAKE KETO POWER BARS

MAKES 12 BARS | PREP TIME: 10 MINUTES PLUS OVERNIGHT TO CHILL

EGG-FREE · PALEO/DAIRY-FREE · VEGAN · BULK PREP · UNDER 30 MINUTES

If you're craving that sweet and salty crunch, these bars are where it's at! Don't be intimidated by the ingredient list; you can add pretty much any variation of low-carb nuts and seeds that you like and they will turn out awesome. You can also use this recipe to make a crumble topping instead of bars. They store great in the refrigerator for weeks.

½ cup pili nuts

½ cup whole hazelnuts

½ cup walnut halves

¼ cup hulled sunflower seeds

¼ cup unsweetened coconut flakes
   or chips

¼ cup hulled hemp seeds

2 tablespoons unsweetened cacao nibs

2 scoops collagen powder (I use
   1 scoop Perfect Keto vanilla collagen
   and 1 scoop Perfect Keto unflavored
   collagen powder)

½ teaspoon ground cinnamon

½ teaspoon sea salt

¼ cup coconut oil, melted

1 teaspoon vanilla extract

Stevia or monk fruit to sweeten
   (optional if you are using unflavored
   collagen powder)

1. Line a 9-inch square baking pan with parchment paper.

2. In a food processor or blender, combine the pili nuts, hazelnuts, walnuts, sunflower seeds, coconut, hemp seeds, cacao nibs, collagen powder, cinnamon, and salt and pulse a few times.

3. Add the coconut oil, vanilla extract, and sweetener (if using). Pulse again until the ingredients are combined. Do not over pulse or it will turn to mush. You want the nuts and seeds to still have some texture.

4. Pour the mixture into the prepared pan and press it into an even layer. Cover with another piece of parchment (or fold over extra from the first piece) and place a heavy pan or dish on top to help press the bars together.

5. Refrigerate overnight and then cut into 12 bars. Store the bars in individual storage bags in the refrigerator for a quick grab-and-go breakfast.

RECIPE TIP: I highly recommend roasting and salting the nuts and seeds beforehand to bring out their flavors.

PER SERVING (1 bar)

Calories: 242; Total Fat: 22g; Protein: 6.5g; Total Carbs: 4.5g; Fiber: 2.5g; Net Carbs: 2g

EASY SKILLET PANCAKES

MAKES 8 PANCAKES | PREP TIME: 5 MINUTES | COOK TIME: 5 MINUTES

NUT-FREE · VEGETARIAN · BULK PREP · UNDER 30 MINUTES

A blender is your best friend for recipes like this one. Keeping a personal-size blender on your counter can come in all sorts of handy between making shakes and smaller servings of these pancakes! This recipe cooks up crisp, just like a regular pancake. Add a few blueberries or strawberries and a heaping spoonful of whipped butter for a delicious breakfast treat.

8 ounces cream cheese

8 eggs

2 tablespoons coconut flour

2 teaspoons baking powder

1 teaspoon ground cinnamon

½ teaspoon vanilla extract

1 teaspoon liquid stevia or sweetener of choice (optional)

2 tablespoons butter

1. In a blender, combine the cream cheese, eggs, coconut flour, baking powder, cinnamon, vanilla, and stevia (if using). Blend until smooth.

2. In a large skillet over medium heat, melt the butter.

3. Use half the mixture to pour four evenly sized pancakes and cook for about a minute, until you see bubbles on top. Flip the pancakes and cook for another minute. Remove from the pan and add more butter or oil to the skillet if needed. Repeat with the remaining batter.

4. Top with butter and eat right away, or freeze the pancakes in a freezer-safe resealable bag with sheets of parchment in between, for up to 1 month.

RECIPE TIP: The coconut flour is dry enough to make these pancakes crispy, so don't substitute a moist flour like almond flour. Choose organic cream cheese, as it generally has fewer carbohydrates than conventional brands.

VARIATION TIP: This batter works to make waffles too. Top it with homemade whipped cream (instructions on page 252) for an extra-indulgent treat.

PER SERVING (1 pancake)

Calories: 179; Total Fat: 15g; Protein: 8g; Total Carbs: 3g; Fiber: 1g; Net Carbs: 2g

QUICK KETO BLENDER MUFFINS

MAKES 12 MUFFINS | PREP TIME: 5 MINUTES | COOK TIME: 25 MINUTES

NUT-FREE · VEGETARIAN · BULK PREP · UNDER 30 MINUTES

These muffins are a staple in my weekly meal prep. They turn out like popovers, very airy and fluffy. Whenever I need a quick breakfast or snack, I pop one of these in the microwave for 15 seconds, add a pat of butter or a teaspoon of nut butter, and I'm good to go. They're perfect for when you're craving a little sweetness without any of the guilt.

Butter, ghee, or coconut oil
   for greasing the pan

6 eggs

8 ounces cream cheese,
   at room temperature

2 scoops flavored collagen powder

1 teaspoon ground cinnamon

1 teaspoon baking powder

Few drops or dash sweetener
   (optional)

1. Preheat the oven to 350°F. Grease a 12-cup muffin pan very well with butter, ghee, or coconut oil. Alternatively, you can use silicone cups or paper muffin liners.

2. In a blender, combine the eggs, cream cheese, collagen powder, cinnamon, baking powder, and sweetener (if using). Blend until well combined and pour the mixture into the muffin cups, dividing equally.

3. Bake for 22 to 25 minutes until the muffins are golden brown on top and firm.

4. Let cool then store in a glass container or plastic bag in the refrigerator for up to 2 weeks or in the freezer for up to 3 months.

5. To serve refrigerated muffins, heat in the microwave for 30 seconds. To serve from frozen, thaw in the refrigerator overnight and then microwave for 30 seconds, or microwave straight from the freezer for 45 to 60 seconds or until heated through.

INGREDIENT TIP: The flavor for these muffins comes mostly from the collagen powder so I recommend using your favorite flavored version. I prefer to use Perfect Keto collagen powder because unlike other protein powders, it has MCT powder in it, which helps with the fat-to-protein ratio. But you can use whichever protein powder you prefer; just remember to adjust the nutritional information.

PER SERVING (1 muffin)

Calories: 120; Total Fat: 10g; Protein: 6g; Total Carbs: 1.5g; Fiber: 0g; Net Carbs: 1.5g

KETO EVERYTHING BAGELS

MAKES 8 BAGELS | PREP TIME: 10 MINUTES | COOK TIME: 15 MINUTES

VEGETARIAN · BULK PREP · UNDER 30 MINUTES

Bagels were a staple for me growing up in Manhattan. If you didn't like bagels, you weren't considered a true New Yorker. These keto bagels are super easy to prepare, store well in the freezer, and unlike regular bagels, have the perfect keto-macronutrient ratio, keeping you full for hours. Add a little bit of cream cheese or butter and you're good to go.

2 cups shredded mozzarella cheese

2 tablespoons labneh cheese
  (or cream cheese)

1½ cups almond flour

1 egg

2 teaspoons baking powder

¼ teaspoon sea salt

1 tablespoon Everything Seasoning
  (page 236)

1. Preheat the oven to 400°F.

2. In a microwave-safe bowl, combine the mozzarella and labneh cheeses. Microwave for 30 seconds, stir, then microwave for another 30 seconds. Stir well. If not melted completely, microwave for another 10 to 20 seconds.

3. Add the almond flour, egg, baking powder, and salt to the bowl and mix well. Form into a dough using a spatula or your hands.

4. Cut the dough into 8 roughly equal pieces and form into balls.

5. Roll each dough ball into a cylinder, then pinch the ends together to seal.

6. Place the dough rings in a nonstick donut pan or arrange them on a parchment paper–lined baking sheet.

7. Sprinkle with the seasoning and bake for 12 to 15 minutes or until golden brown.

8. Store in plastic bags in the freezer and defrost overnight in the refrigerator. Reheat in the oven or toaster for a quick grab-and-go breakfast.

INGREDIENT TIP: Labneh cheese is a Greek-style kefir cheese that is a hidden gem in many grocery stores. It's a close cousin to cream cheese with a slight tangy flavor similar to sour cream.

PER SERVING (1 bagel)

Calories: 241; Total Fat: 19g; Protein: 12g; Total Carbs: 5.5g; Fiber: 2.5g; Net Carbs: 3g

KETO BISCUITS AND GRAVY

SERVES 8 | PREP TIME: 10 MINUTES | COOK TIME: 15 MINUTES

NUT-FREE OPTION · BULK PREP · UNDER 30 MINUTES

These biscuits and gravy are perfect for any day of the week. You can whip them up for a quick weekend brunch or make them ahead of time for an easy breakfast, lunch, or even dinner during the week. Flavor the biscuits any way you like by adding different types of cheese, spices, and chopped chives, jalapeños, parsley, or anything else to bump up the flavor.

FOR THE BISCUITS

2 cups almond flour (or ½ cup coconut flour)

2 teaspoons baking powder

½ teaspoon sea salt

½ teaspoon garlic powder

½ teaspoon onion powder

½ cup shredded Cheddar cheese (about 2 ounces) (optional)

3 tablespoons cold butter, cut into small pieces

2 eggs

¼ cup sour cream (½ cup if using coconut flour)

FOR THE GRAVY

12 ounces breakfast sausage or ground pork

⅓ cup heavy (whipping) cream

2 ounces cream cheese

Pinch sea salt

Pinch freshly ground black pepper

TO MAKE THE BISCUITS

1. Preheat the oven to 400°F and line a baking sheet with parchment paper.

2. In a medium bowl, whisk together the almond flour (or coconut flour), baking powder, salt, garlic powder, onion powder, and Cheddar (if using). If adding other herbs or spices, do so at this time.

3. Add the butter, eggs, and sour cream. Mix just until combined (do not overmix or the biscuits will become dense).

4. Form the dough into 8 biscuits and place them on the prepared baking sheet. Bake for 12 to 15 minutes or until golden brown.

5. Store the biscuits in an airtight container or freezer-safe resealable bag for up to 3 months. To serve, reheat from frozen in the oven or microwave for 1 to 1½ minutes.

TO MAKE THE GRAVY

1. In a medium skillet over medium-high heat, cook the sausage until browned, 5 to 7 minutes.

2. Add the cream, cream cheese, salt, and pepper and cook for another 5 minutes until melted and well combined.

3. Serve over the biscuits and store any remainder in the refrigerator for up to 1 week or in the freezer for up to 2 months.

INGREDIENT TIP: Using breakfast sausage will give the gravy more flavor, but make sure to read the ingredient label on your breakfast sausage to make sure there's no added sugar or carbs. To be safe, use ground pork and add your own spices for flavor.

RECIPE TIP: If making coconut flour biscuits, they will be slighter smaller than the almond flour biscuits when divided into 8. You can divide them into 6 instead, but remember to adjust the nutritional information below.

PER SERVING
(1 almond flour biscuit with cheese)

Calories: 269; Total Fat: 23g; Protein: 9g; Total Carbs: 6.5g; Fiber: 3g; Net Carbs: 3.5g

PER SERVING
(1 coconut flour biscuit with cheese)

Calories: 139; Total Fat: 11g; Protein: 5g; Total Carbs: 5g; Fiber: 2.5g; Net Carbs: 2.5g

PER SERVING (about ⅓ cup gravy)

Calories: 189; Total Fat: 17g; Protein: 8g; Total Carbs: 1g; Fiber: 0g; Net Carbs: 1g

NOT YOUR AVERAGE BOILED EGGS

SERVES 5 | PREP TIME: 10 MINUTES PLUS SOAKING TIME | COOK TIME: 10 MINUTES

NUT-FREE · PALEO/DAIRY-FREE · VEGETARIAN · BULK PREP

Hard-boiled eggs are a staple in my house because they're so easy and convenient for any meal or snack. This recipe is my take on "soy eggs" and it's an amazing alternative to traditional boiled eggs because it adds both sweet and salty flavor to them. They store in the refrigerator for weeks and you can continue to add eggs to the jar as you eat them. Just make sure to use an airtight container and shake it well every few days.

FOR THE BOILED EGGS

10 eggs

1 tablespoon coconut vinegar
   or apple cider vinegar

FOR THE SAUCE

1½ cups water

2 tablespoons liquid aminos or tamari

2 tablespoons coconut aminos

2 tablespoons coconut vinegar
   or apple cider vinegar

1 teaspoon minced fresh garlic
   or garlic powder

1 teaspoon minced fresh ginger
   or ground ginger

1 teaspoon sea salt

½ teaspoon freshly ground
   black pepper

TO MAKE THE BOILED EGGS

1. Place the eggs in a medium pot and add enough cold water to cover them. Add a splash of vinegar (this makes the eggs easier to peel) and bring to a boil. When the water boils, remove the pot from the heat, cover, and let sit for 10 minutes.

2. Meanwhile, fill a large bowl with water and ice. When the eggs are done, transfer them to the ice bath for another 10 minutes.

3. Peel the eggs and set them aside.

TO MAKE THE SAUCE

1. In a large storage bowl with a lid, whisk together the water, liquid aminos, coconut aminos, vinegar, garlic, ginger, salt, and pepper. Alternatively, you can divide the ingredients in half and add to two large mason jars with lids.

2. Place the peeled eggs in the sauce. Cover and refrigerate. The longer the eggs soak up the sauce, the more flavorful they will be.

INGREDIENT TIP: Liquid aminos are made from non-GMO soybeans. They are gluten-free and are an excellent alternative to soy sauce or tamari. Coconut aminos are similar but made from coconut sap. They are soy-free and have a slightly nuttier and sweeter taste. They can both be found in most grocery stores or purchased online.

PER SERVING (2 eggs)

Calories: 144; Total Fat: 10g; Protein: 12g; Total Carbs: 1.5g; Fiber: 0g; Net Carbs: 1.5g

CHEESY BACON GRAB-AND-GO EGG MUFFINS

MAKES 12 MUFFINS | PREP TIME: 10 MINUTES | COOK TIME: 20 MINUTES

NUT-FREE · PALEO/DAIRY-FREE OPTION · BULK PREP · UNDER 30 MINUTES

Egg muffins are the perfect grab-and-go breakfast (or lunch) for any day of the week. I prep mine on Sunday nights and store them in an airtight glass container in the refrigerator for the entire week. Just pop them in the microwave for 30 seconds to a minute, add a dash hot sauce or salt and pepper and you've got a one-minute breakfast.

Butter, ghee, or coconut oil,
   for greasing

12 bacon slices

12 eggs

1 teaspoon garlic powder

½ teaspoon sea salt

¼ teaspoon freshly ground
   black pepper

1 cup shredded sharp Cheddar cheese

1. Preheat the oven to 350°F. Grease a muffin pan very well with butter, ghee, or coconut oil. Alternatively, you can use silicone cups or parchment paper muffin liners.

2. In a large skillet over medium-high heat, cook the bacon in batches until crisp, 5 to 7 minutes, and let drain on a paper towel.

3. Crack the eggs into a large bowl. Add the garlic powder, salt, and pepper and whisk to combine.

4. Divide the egg mixture equally among the muffin cups. Crumble one slice of bacon over the top of each muffin cup. Sprinkle the cheese on top, dividing equally.

5. Bake for 12 to 15 minutes or until the eggs are firm and slightly golden brown along the edges.

6. Divide the muffins into glass containers or plastic bags and store in the refrigerator for the week or freeze for up to 2 months.

7. To serve, reheat in the microwave for 30 to 45 seconds.

VARIATION TIP: Swap the bacon and Cheddar for any other meat or cheese of choice (e.g., ground sausage, ground beef, goat cheese, feta cheese, etc.).

MAKE IT PALEO/DAIRY-FREE: Add extra meat or vegetables instead of cheese.

PER SERVING (2 muffins)

Calories: 324; Total Fat: 24g; Protein: 25g; Total Carbs: 2g; Fiber: 0g; Net Carbs: 2g

SAUSAGE, SPINACH, AND GOAT CHEESE BREAKFAST CASSEROLE

MAKES 10 SQUARES | PREP TIME: 10 MINUTES | COOK TIME: 40 MINUTES

NUT-FREE · PALEO/DAIRY-FREE OPTION · BULK PREP

This is one of my favorite Sunday meal prep recipes for breakfast or lunch during the week. It's quick, easy, and stores very well in the refrigerator or freezer. Pop it in the microwave for about a minute and top it with your favorite hot sauce or salsa. Feel free to mix up the meat, veggies, and cheese for alternative options.

Butter or coconut oil, for greasing

1 pound breakfast sausage
 or ground pork

1 (10-ounce) package frozen spinach,
 thawed and squeezed to remove
 excess liquid

12 eggs

½ cup heavy (whipping) cream

1 teaspoon sea salt

½ teaspoon freshly ground
 black pepper

5 ounces goat cheese, crumbled

1. Preheat the oven to 400°F and grease a 9-by-13-inch baking dish.

2. In a medium bowl, break up the sausage into small pieces. Add the spinach and mix well. Spread the mixture over the bottom of the prepared baking dish.

3. In a large bowl, whisk together the eggs, cream, salt, and pepper. Slowly pour the egg mixture over the sausage and spinach and then top with the cheese.

4. Bake for 30 to 40 minutes until fluffy and set.

5. Let cool and then cut into 10 squares. Refrigerate portions for the week in a glass container or resealable plastic bag and freeze the rest for up to 3 months. To serve, reheat in the microwave for 1 minute if previously thawed in the refrigerator overnight or 2 minutes if frozen.

MAKE IT PALEO/DAIRY-FREE: Substitute unsweetened hemp, almond, or cashew milk for the cream. Omit the cheese.

INGREDIENT TIP: Using breakfast sausage will give this dish more flavor, but make sure to check the ingredients of the sausage for added sugar or carbs and choose one with a higher fat-to-protein ratio. To be safe, use ground pork and add your own spices for flavor.

PER SERVING (1 square)

Calories: 322; Total Fat: 26g; Protein: 19g; Total Carbs: 3g; Fiber: 1g; Net Carbs: 2g

BAE BREAKFAST BOWL

SERVES 1 | PREP TIME: 5 MINUTES | COOK TIME: 10 MINUTES

NUT-FREE · PALEO/DAIRY-FREE · UNDER 30 MINUTES

This is one of my favorite weekday breakfasts. It's super quick and hits the spot every time. If you're short on time in the morning, you can easily make this a "bulk prep" option by cooking the bacon ahead of time and storing it in the refrigerator. Instead of making fried eggs, make hard-boiled or soft-boiled eggs and store those, as well. Reheat the bacon and eggs in the microwave for quick assembly.

2 bacon slices

½ medium avocado, pitted

2 eggs

Pinch sea salt

Pinch freshly ground black pepper

Dash hot sauce

1. Cook the bacon in a skillet over medium-high heat until crisp, 5 to 7 minutes. Transfer the bacon to a paper towel, leaving the grease in the skillet.

2. Add the eggs to the pan and fry to your liking.

3. To assemble the bowl, scoop the avocado half out of its peel and cut it in half lengthwise. Place it on the bottom of the bowl and sprinkle with salt and pepper. Top with the fried eggs and then crumble the bacon over the top. Add the hot sauce and enjoy.

VARIATION TIP: Substitute ground sausage or meat of your choice for the bacon. Add some cheese on top for extra flavor.

PER SERVING

Calories: 360; Total Fat: 28g; Protein: 19g; Total Carbs: 8g; Fiber: 5g; Net Carbs: 3g

EASY CHEESY SAUSAGE BALLS

MAKES 30 BALLS | PREP TIME: 10 MINUTES | COOK TIME: 20 MINUTES

EGG-FREE OPTION · NUT-FREE · BULK PREP · UNDER 30 MINUTES

These sausage balls are simple to make yet bursting with flavor. I usually make one batch at the beginning of the week, freeze half of them and store the rest in the refrigerator for a quick breakfast or snack.

1 pound ground sausage

1½ cups shredded Cheddar cheese

1 egg

1 teaspoon sea salt

½ teaspoon freshly ground
black pepper

1. Preheat the oven to 375°F and line two large baking sheets with parchment paper or silicone mats.

2. In a large bowl, mix together the sausage, Cheddar, egg, salt, and pepper.

3. Using a tablespoon, scoop the mixture onto the prepared baking sheet and form the scoops into balls. You should end up with 30 sausage balls in total.

4. Bake for 18 to 20 minutes or until browned.

5. Let cool for 20 to 30 minutes and then store in the refrigerator for up to 1 week or in the freezer for up to 2 months.

INGREDIENT TIP: Choose your favorite sausage, but make sure to check the ingredient label for added sugar or carbs. You can also use ground beef or pork and season with spices of your choice.

EGG-FREE OPTION: You can replace the egg with ¼ cup crushed pork rinds or leave it out altogether.

PER SERVING (2 sausage balls)

Calories: 148; Total Fat: 12g; Protein: 9g; Total Carbs: 1g; Fiber: 0g; Net Carbs: 1g

BACON-WRAPPED WESTERN QUICHE TARTS

MAKES 12 QUICHE TARTS | PREP TIME: 10 MINUTES | COOK TIME: 20 MINUTES

NUT-FREE · PALEO/DAIRY-FREE OPTION · BULK PREP · UNDER 30 MINUTES

These tarts make a perfect grab-and-go breakfast. Make them on Sunday and enjoy them all week. They check off all the savory flavor boxes on your taste buds and keep you full all day long.

12 bacon slices

8 eggs

⅓ cup heavy (whipping) cream

1 cup shredded Cheddar cheese

¼ cup finely diced red bell pepper

¼ cup finely diced green bell pepper

¼ cup finely diced yellow onion

1. Preheat the oven to 375°F.

2. Line each cup of a 12-cup muffin tin with a slice of bacon around the edges and then bake for about 10 minutes until browned but not crisp.

3. In a large bowl, whisk together the eggs and cream. Add the Cheddar, red and green bell peppers, and onion and mix well.

4. Pour the egg mixture into the bacon-lined muffin cups, filling each about three-quarters full.

5. Bake for about 20 minutes until the muffins are golden brown and fully cooked. They should be spongy but not soft in the middle. Use a spoon to lift them from the pan.

6. Store in an airtight container in the refrigerator for up to 1 week.

MAKE IT PALEO/DAIRY-FREE: You can make this recipe without cream or cheese. Simply add 2 more eggs.

VARIATION TIP: Add flavorful mix-ins like crumbled sausage or diced pepperoni.

PER SERVING (1 quiche tart)

Calories: 154; Total Fat: 12g; Protein: 10g; Total Carbs: 1.5g; Fiber: 0g; Net Carbs: 1.5g

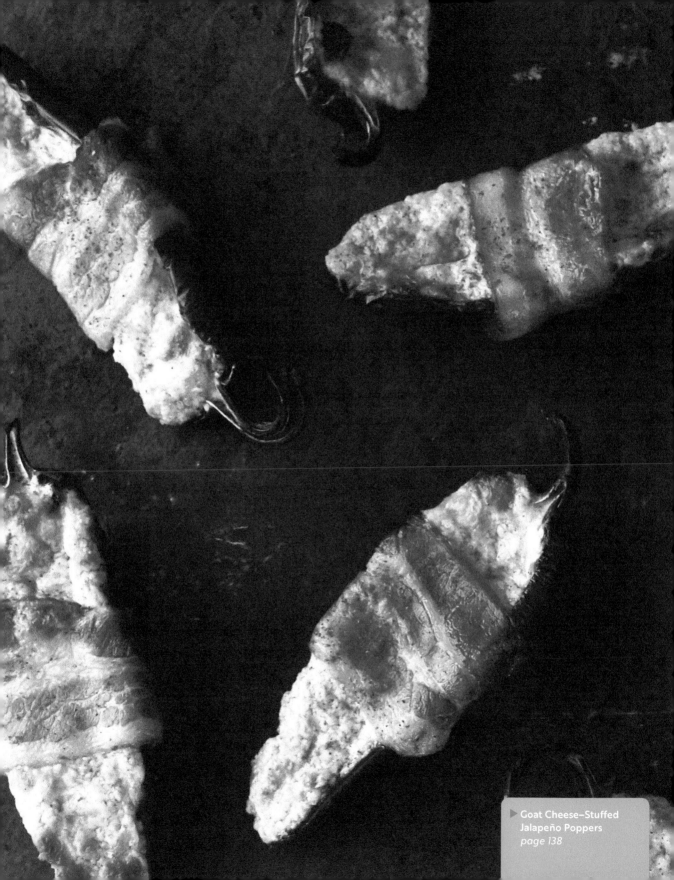

▶ Goat Cheese–Stuffed
Jalapeño Poppers
page 138

6

Appetizers and Snacks

AVOCADO FETA DIP

SERVES 8 | PREP TIME: 15 MINUTES PLUS 2 HOURS TO CHILL

EGG-FREE · NUT-FREE · VEGETARIAN

This is the most delicious, quick, and easy dip that can be whipped up for any occasion—party appetizers, side dish, or even as a topping for a salad or omelet. You can even prepare most of it the day before by combining everything except the avocado, and just add that a few hours before serving. Serve with celery, cucumber, Keto Crackers (page 136), pork rinds, salami, or cheese crisps.

2 avocados, diced

2 Roma tomatoes, chopped

¼ medium red onion, finely chopped (about ½ cup)

2 garlic cloves, minced

2 tablespoons chopped fresh parsley (or cilantro)

2 tablespoons olive oil or avocado oil

2 tablespoons red wine vinegar

1 tablespoon freshly squeezed lemon or lime juice

½ teaspoon sea salt

¼ teaspoon freshly ground black pepper

8 ounces feta cheese, crumbled

1. In a large bowl, gently stir together the avocados, tomatoes, onion, garlic, and parsley.

2. In a small bowl, whisk together the oil, vinegar, lemon juice, salt, and pepper. Pour the mixture over the avocado mixture. Fold in the cheese.

3. Cover and let chill in the refrigerator for 1 to 2 hours before serving.

VARIATION TIP: Not a fan of feta? Swap in a different cheese that you like. I sometimes make this recipe with crumbled goat cheese and it's delicious.

PER SERVING (½ cup dip)

Calories: 190; Total Fat: 16g; Protein: 6g; Total Carbs: 5.5g; Fiber: 3g; Net Carbs: 2.5g

SOUTHERN PIMENTO CHEESE DIP

SERVES 10 | PREP TIME: 5 MINUTES PLUS 2 HOURS TO CHILL

NUT-FREE · VEGETARIAN

It's hard to go wrong with cheese dip when you're trying to please a crowd or just looking for some yummy comfort food. This pimento cheese dip takes 5 minutes to whip together, but I recommend making it the night before so it can sit in the refrigerator to let the flavors come together. Serve with celery, cucumber, Keto Crackers (page 136), pork rinds, or salami, or use as a topping for salad.

8 ounces cream cheese, at room temperature

1 cup shredded sharp Cheddar cheese

1 cup shredded pepper Jack cheese

⅓ cup mayonnaise

1 (4-ounce) jar pimentos, diced

1 teaspoon garlic powder

1 teaspoon onion powder

¼ teaspoon cayenne pepper

Pinch sea salt

Pinch freshly ground black pepper

1. In a large bowl, combine the cream cheese, Cheddar, pepper Jack, mayonnaise, pimentos, garlic powder, onion powder, and cayenne. Beat together using an electric mixer. Season with salt and pepper and beat again until well combined.

2. Chill in the refrigerator for a few hours (or overnight) to let the flavors set.

INGREDIENT TIP: Make sure to use mayonnaise that's made with healthy oils such as avocado or olive oil. I like the Primal Kitchen or Chosen Foods brands. You could also make your own from scratch.

PER SERVING (about ⅓ cup dip)

Calories: 225; Total Fat: 21g; Protein: 7g; Total Carbs: 2g; Fiber: 0g; Net Carbs: 2g

KETO CRACKERS

MAKES 36 CRACKERS | PREP TIME: 10 MINUTES | COOK TIME: 15 MINUTES

NUT-FREE OPTION · PALEO/DAIRY-FREE · VEGETARIAN · UNDER 30 MINUTES

These crackers are versatile and great to serve alongside any dip or crumble over a hearty bowl of keto soup. You can flavor them however you like by simply adding different herbs and spices to the dough. It's hard to go wrong with this simple, quick, and tasty Keto Cracker.

1 batch Keto Dough (page 242; traditional, dairy-free, or nut-free)

1 tablespoon your choice "In a Hurry" Spice Blend (page 236)

½ teaspoon sea salt

1. Preheat the oven to 400°F and line one large (or two medium) baking sheets with parchment paper or a silicone mat.

2. Prepare the dough, mixing in your spices of choice when prompted. If you are using an already prepared dough, thaw overnight in the refrigerator. Once defrosted and warmed to a workable consistency, knead in the spices and sea salt until well combined.

3. Place the dough between two pieces of parchment paper and roll it out to a thickness of about ⅛ to ¼ inch. Remove the top piece of parchment and, using a sharp knife or pizza cutter, cut the dough into 1-inch squares.

4. Arrange the squares on the prepared baking sheet(s) and bake for 10 to 15 minutes until golden brown. Let cool for 5 minutes or until crisp.

5. These crackers are best eaten right away, but they can be stored for up to 1 week in the refrigerator. Reheat in a 400°F oven for about 10 minutes before serving.

RECIPE TIP: If the dough is slightly sticky or falling apart when you are trying to cut the crackers, place it in the refrigerator for 5 to 10 minutes to firm up.

PER SERVING
(1 Traditional Keto Cracker)

Calories: 39; Total Fat: 3g; Protein: 2g; Total Carbs: 1g; Fiber: 0.5g; Net Carbs: 0.5g

PER SERVING
(1 Paleo/Dairy-Free Keto Cracker)

Calories: 39; Total Fat: 3g; Protein: 2g; Total Carbs: 1g; Fiber: 0.5g; Net Carbs: 0.5g

PER SERVING (1 Nut-Free Keto Cracker)

Calories: 28; Total Fat: 2g; Protein: 1.5g; Total Carbs: 1g; Fiber: 0.5g; Net Carbs: 0.5g

PIZZA BAGEL BITES

SERVES 16 | PREP TIME: 10 MINUTES | COOK TIME: 20 MINUTES

VEGETARIAN OPTION · BULK PREP · UNDER 30 MINUTES

When I was a kid, I loved those mini frozen bagel bites that were so easy to pop in the oven and then into your mouth for a quick snack. Just like the traditional bagel bites, these are super easy to throw together and great for bringing to parties or for when you're craving a few bites of yummy pizza. Make the dough ahead of time and you've got a quick and easy keto crowd-pleaser.

1 batch Keto Dough (page 242) with 2 tablespoons Italian seasoning mixed in before kneading

½ cup low-sugar tomato sauce

1 cup shredded mozzarella cheese

32 pepperoni slices (optional)

1. Preheat the oven to 400°F. Line one large (or two medium) baking sheets with parchment paper or a silicone mat.

2. Split the dough into 16 golf ball–size portions (each should weigh about 1 ounce). Place the dough balls on the prepared baking sheet(s) and press down gently to form small disks.

3. Bake for 12 to 15 minutes until golden brown.

4. Remove from the oven and let cool for 5 minutes. Once cooled, cut each disk in half and return to the baking sheet.

5. Top with a spoonful of tomato sauce, a sprinkle of cheese, 1 pepperoni slice (if using), and another small sprinkle of cheese.

6. Return to the oven for about 5 minutes until the cheese is melted.

VARIATION TIP: You can use any toppings that you normally like on pizza. Replace the tomato sauce with pesto or white garlic sauce and top with chopped artichokes, shredded chicken, sausage, or any other pizza toppings.

PER SERVING (2 bites)

Calories: 154; Total Fat: 12g; Protein: 8g; Total Carbs: 3.5g; Fiber: 1.5g; Net Carbs: 2g

GOAT CHEESE–STUFFED JALAPEÑO POPPERS

SERVES 8 | PREP TIME: 15 MINUTES | COOK TIME: 20 MINUTES

EGG-FREE · NUT-FREE

Traditional jalapeño poppers are breaded, deep-fried, and stuffed with cream cheese. I promise, this version is just as good, if not better! Replace the breading with bacon and substitute goat cheese for the cream cheese and you've got yourself a keto flavor bomb that hits all those cravings—crunchy, creamy, spicy, and salty.

1 (5-ounce) package goat cheese, at room temperature

¼ cup shredded white Cheddar cheese

1 teaspoon paprika

½ teaspoon garlic powder

½ teaspoon onion powder

½ teaspoon sea salt

½ teaspoon freshly ground black pepper

8 jalapeño peppers

8 bacon slices

1. Preheat the oven to 400°F and line a baking sheet with aluminum foil. Put a baking rack on the sheet.

2. In a medium bowl, mix together the goat cheese, Cheddar, paprika, garlic powder, onion powder, salt, and pepper.

3. Cut the jalapeños in half lengthwise and scoop out the seeds. Fill each half generously with the cheese mixture.

4. Cut the bacon slices in half to make 16 individual pieces. Wrap each jalapeño half with one piece of bacon and place on the baking rack.

5. Cook for 15 to 20 minutes until the bacon begins to crisp.

6. Broil for an additional 2 to 3 minutes until the cheese is bubbly and slightly browned.

VARIATION TIP: If you're not a big fan of jalapeños, you can use baby bell peppers instead, preparing them the same way. They will lend a slight sweetness to the poppers.

PER SERVING (2 poppers)

Calories: 121; Total Fat: 9g; Protein: 8g; Total Carbs: 2g; Fiber: 0.5g; Net Carbs: 1.5g

DILL DEVILED EGGS

MAKES 12 DEVILED EGG HALVES | PREP TIME: 5 MINUTES

NUT-FREE · PALEO/DAIRY-FREE · VEGETARIAN · UNDER 30 MINUTES

Deviled eggs are an amazing ketogenic snack, and they work especially well for parties when you want to bring something you can eat, but you don't want to bring "diet food." You can cook your hard-boiled eggs however you like or look at the Not Your Average Boiled Eggs recipe (page 124) to see my preferred method.

6 hard-boiled eggs

3 tablespoons mayonnaise

¼ teaspoon dried dill or 1 teaspoon chopped fresh dill

Pinch ground yellow mustard seed

Sea salt

1. Slice the hard-boiled eggs in half lengthwise. Remove the yolks from the whites and put them in a small bowl.

2. To the egg yolks, add the mayonnaise, dill, and mustard seed and mash everything together until smooth. Season with salt.

3. Spoon the yolk mixture into the egg whites or use a resealable plastic bag with one corner snipped off to pipe the filling into the egg whites.

4. Store in an airtight container in the refrigerator for up to 5 days.

INGREDIENT TIP: Use mayonnaise that's made with healthy oils such as avocado or olive oil. Primal Kitchen and Chosen Foods brands are great options.

VARIATION TIP: Dill is just the tip of the deviled egg iceberg. Try it with fresh thyme, crumbled bacon, chopped scallions, crumbled blue cheese, or chopped sun-dried tomatoes.

PER SERVING (2 halves)

Calories: 116; Total Fat: 10g; Protein: 6g; Total Carbs: 0.6g; Fiber: 0g; Net Carbs: 0.6g

EASY BACON-BROCCOLI SALAD

SERVES 10 | PREP TIME: 15 MINUTES | COOK TIME: 10 MINUTES

NUT-FREE · PALEO/DAIRY-FREE OPTION · BULK PREP · UNDER 30 MINUTES

I was the kid growing up who actually enjoyed eating broccoli. Weird, I know. But even if you're not a fan of broccoli, this recipe is sure to change your mind. The combination of the crunchy bacon and broccoli paired with the creamy, tangy dressing is amazing. Enjoy it alone as a snack or serve alongside a tasty protein for lunch or dinner. It stores great in the refrigerator all week.

6 bacon slices

2 (12-ounce) bags raw broccoli florets (about 10 cups)

1 cup shredded sharp Cheddar cheese

¼ cup hulled sunflower seeds, roasted and salted

1 tablespoon Everything Seasoning (page 236)

Reserved bacon grease (about 1 ounce)

⅓ cup mayonnaise

½ cup sour cream

1 tablespoon apple cider vinegar

Sea salt

1. In a large skillet over medium-high heat, cook the bacon until crisp, 5 to 7 minutes. Remove the bacon to a paper towel, reserving the bacon grease for the dressing.

2. Meanwhile, in a large bowl, combine the broccoli florets, Cheddar, sunflower seeds, and seasoning. Mix well.

3. To make the dressing, in a medium bowl, whisk together the reserved bacon grease, mayonnaise, sour cream, and vinegar.

4. Pour the dressing over the broccoli mixture and toss until well combined.

5. Taste and season with salt.

6. Serve immediately or store in the refrigerator for up to 1 week.

MAKE IT PALEO/DAIRY-FREE: Replace the cheese with a few more bacon slices and use an extra ⅓ cup mayonnaise in place of the sour cream.

VARIATION TIP: If you're not in the mood to make the dressing, just use about a half-cup of your favorite low-carb dressing, such as ranch or Caesar.

PER SERVING (about 1½ cups)

Calories: 214; Total Fat: 18g; Protein: 8g; Total Carbs: 5.5g; Fiber: 2g; Net Carbs: 3.5g

KETO ANTIPASTO

SERVES 12 | PREP TIME: 20 MINUTES

EGG-FREE · NUT-FREE · BULK PREP · UNDER 30 MINUTES

This recipe was inspired by one of my favorite areas in San Diego, Little Italy. Many people think that it's impossible to eat keto at an Italian restaurant, but if you stick with the meats and cheeses, you'll be fine. Most Italian restaurants serve amazing antipasto salads or platters with delicious gourmet meats and cheeses. This is my version that can be enjoyed as an appetizer or snack or made into a perfect keto meal by tossing with a few cups of lettuce and another drizzle of olive oil.

8 ounces soppressata salami, diced

5 ounces Calabrese salami, diced

4 ounces sharp provolone or white Cheddar cheese, diced

4 ounces mozzarella, diced

4 celery stalks, diced

¼ medium red onion, finely chopped (about ½ cup)

24 large green olives (or 35 medium), pitted and chopped

10 pepperoncini peppers, diced

¼ cup fresh basil, chopped

1 tablespoon Italian seasoning

2 tablespoons olive oil

2 tablespoons red wine vinegar

1 teaspoon balsamic vinegar

1 teaspoon Dijon mustard

Sea salt

Freshly ground black pepper

PER SERVING (about ⅓ cup)

Calories: 206; Total Fat: 16g; Protein: 12g; Total Carbs: 3.5g; Fiber: 0.5g; Net Carbs: 3g

1. In a large bowl, combine the soppressata, Calabrese, provolone, mozzarella, celery, onion, olives, peppers, basil, and Italian seasoning. Mix until well combined.

2. In a small bowl, whisk together the olive oil, red wine vinegar, balsamic vinegar, and mustard. Add salt and pepper.

3. Pour the dressing over the meat and cheese mixture and stir well.

4. Serve immediately or transfer to an airtight container and store in the refrigerator for up to 1 week or in the freezer for up to 3 months.

INGREDIENT TIP: Soppressata is an Italian dried salami that is usually found in the gourmet meat and cheese section of the grocery store. Calabrese is a mildly spicy pork salami usually found sliced in the meat section of the grocery store. Feel free to swap soppressata for any other hard salami and Calabrese for pepperoni or other salami of choice.

CRISPY WINGS THREE WAYS

SERVES 6 | PREP TIME: 5 MINUTES | COOK TIME: 60 MINUTES

EGG-FREE · NUT-FREE · PALEO/DAIRY-FREE

Wings are an easy, budget-friendly option for serving at parties or enjoying for a simple meal paired with a side salad or vegetable. Of course, having a tasty sauce to toss your wings in is very important, which is why I've provided three different keto sauces that are easy to prepare and super tasty.

FOR THE WINGS

3 pounds chicken wings (about 20 to 24 drumettes/wingettes, depending on size)

2 tablespoons baking powder

2 teaspoons sea salt, divided

1. Preheat the oven to 250°F and line a large baking sheet (or two) with aluminum foil and a baking rack. Grease or spray the rack with oil to prevent the chicken from sticking.

2. Pat the wings dry with a paper towel and place in a paper or plastic bag. Add the baking powder and salt and shake until the wings are completely coated.

3. Place the wings on the baking rack and cook for 30 minutes.

4. After 30 minutes, raise the oven temperature to 425°F and cook for an additional 30 to 40 minutes until crisp.

5. Remove from the oven and let cool for 5 minutes.

6. Toss the wings in your chosen sauce and serve.

PER SERVING (3 to 4 wings)

Calories: 297; Total Fat: 21g; Protein: 27g; Total Carbs: 0g; Fiber: 0g; Net Carbs: 0g

Buffalo Sauce

½ cup Frank's RedHot Sauce

2 tablespoons butter, melted

1 teaspoon garlic powder

Sea salt

Freshly ground black pepper

In a large bowl, whisk together the hot sauce, butter, garlic powder, salt, and pepper.

PER SERVING (3 to 4 wings)

Calories: 333; Total Fat: 25g; Protein: 27g; Total Carbs: 0g; Fiber: 0g; Net Carbs: 0g

Garlic and Parmesan Sauce

¼ cup butter

3 garlic cloves, minced

1 teaspoon onion powder

½ to 1 teaspoon red pepper flakes

1 tablespoon chopped fresh parsley

½ cup freshly grated Parmesan cheese

Sea salt

Freshly ground black pepper

1. In a small saucepan, melt the butter over medium heat. Add the garlic and cook for 3 minutes.
2. Remove the pan from the heat and add the onion powder, red pepper flakes, parsley, Parmesan, salt, and pepper. Stir to mix well.

PER SERVING (3 to 4 wings)

Calories: 403; Total Fat: 31g; Protein: 30g; Total Carbs: 1g; Fiber: 0.2g; Net Carbs: 0.8g

CONTINUED

Sweet and Spicy Sauce

2 tablespoons butter or ghee

3 garlic cloves, minced

2 tablespoons coconut aminos

2 tablespoons coconut vinegar
or rice wine vinegar

½ tablespoon chili paste

½ cup water

Dash monk fruit or sweetener
of choice

1 tablespoon sesame seeds (optional)

1. In a small saucepan, melt the butter over medium heat. Add the garlic and cook for 3 minutes.

2. Add the coconut aminos, vinegar, chili paste, and water. Bring to a boil, then lower the heat to medium and simmer for 10 minutes until thickened.

3. Remove from the heat and sweeten with monk fruit. Add the sesame seeds (if using).

INGREDIENT TIP: Chili paste can be found in the international aisle of most grocery stores. You can also use harissa paste or make a quick paste by mixing or muddling together ½ tablespoon of red pepper flakes with ½ tablespoon of oil.

RECIPE TIP: These sauces are great for using in other dishes, too. Use them to top roasted vegetables, meats, and fish.

PER SERVING (3 to 4 wings)

Calories: 349; Total Fat: 25g; Protein: 29g; Total Carbs: 2g; Fiber: 0.2g; Net Carbs: 1.8g

LOADED BACON AND CHEDDAR CHEESE BALLS

MAKES 16 BALLS | 8 SERVINGS | PREP TIME: 10 MINUTES

EGG-FREE · NUT-FREE · BULK PREP · UNDER 30 MINUTES

Think baked potato but replace the potato with cream cheese. Although cheese is lower in carbohydrates than most foods, it can get pretty bulky, so these cheese balls have less cheese and more bacon. These are easy to pick up and pop in your mouth, and they're "loaded" with all the fixin's.

7 bacon slices, cooked until crisp, cooled, and crumbled

1 tablespoon chopped chives

8 ounces cream cheese

1½ cups finely shredded Cheddar cheese

½ teaspoon smoked paprika

1 teaspoon onion powder

½ teaspoon sea salt

Olive oil or butter, for greasing

1. Line a plate or storage container with parchment paper.
2. In a small bowl, toss together the crumbled bacon and chives and set aside.
3. In a food processor or blender, mix together the cream cheese, Cheddar, paprika, onion powder, and salt.
4. Grease your hands with olive oil or butter to avoid sticking, and form 16 balls of cheese. Roll each ball in the bacon and chive "batter" as you go, and set them on the prepared plate or storage container.
5. Serve right away, or store in an airtight container in the refrigerator for up to 5 days.

VARIATION TIP: Feel free to add more bacon, substitute goat cheese for the cream cheese, or add some cayenne pepper for a little kick.

PER SERVING (2 cheese balls)

Calories: 228; Total Fat: 20g; Protein: 10g; Total Carbs: 2g; Fiber: 0g; Net Carbs: 2g

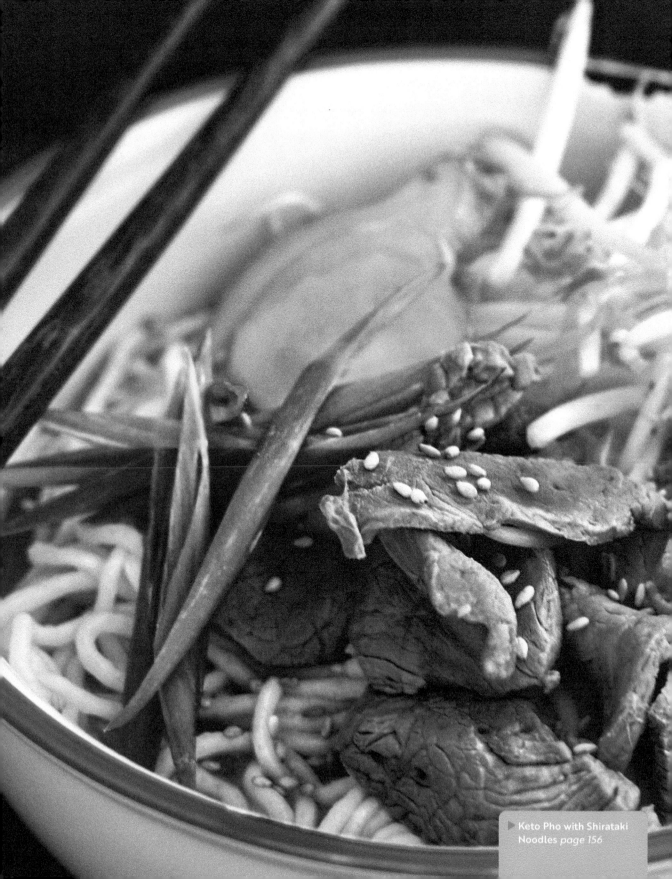

▶ Keto Pho with Shirataki
Noodles *page 156*

7

Salads, Soups, and Stews

SPECIAL SAUCE COBB SALAD

SERVES 4 | PREP TIME: 15 MINUTES | COOK TIME: 10 MINUTES

NUT-FREE · PALEO/DAIRY-FREE OPTION · BULK PREP · UNDER 30 MINUTES

Two of my favorite things in one meal: the "special sauce" from a Big Mac, and Cobb salad. Sounds weird but I promise it's tasty and will bring back childhood memories. The dressing is tangy and sweet and can be used as a dipping sauce for veggies or other keto-friendly snacks. To make this as close to a real Big Mac as possible, swap the bacon and eggs for cooked and seasoned ground beef.

4 bacon slices

¼ cup mayonnaise

½ teaspoon coconut vinegar or apple cider vinegar

¼ teaspoon paprika

¼ teaspoon garlic powder

¼ teaspoon onion powder

¼ teaspoon sea salt

Dash monk fruit or sweetener of choice

8 cherry tomatoes, halved

4 hard-boiled eggs, sliced

1 cup shredded sharp Cheddar cheese

8 cups chopped romaine lettuce or spinach

1. In a large skillet over medium-high heat, cook the bacon until crisp, 5 to 7 minutes. Remove the bacon to a paper towel.

2. While the bacon is cooking, prepare the dressing. In a medium bowl, whisk together the mayonnaise, vinegar, paprika, garlic powder, onion powder, salt, and sweetener.

3. To serve immediately, divide the lettuce among four serving bowls. To each bowl, add 4 tomato halves, 1 sliced egg, ¼ cup Cheddar, 1 crumbled bacon slice, and 1 tablespoon of dressing. Mix well.

4. To assemble and store for future meals, divide and layer the components in four quart-sized, wide-mouth mason jars, adding the ingredients in the following order: 1 tablespoon of dressing, 4 tomato halves, 1 sliced egg, ¼ cup Cheddar, 2 cups of romaine, and top with 1 crumbled bacon slice. Secure the lid tightly and store in the refrigerator. To serve, shake well and empty the jar into a bowl—or you can eat the salad right out of the jar!

MAKE IT PALEO/DAIRY-FREE: Ditch the cheese and add 1 tablespoon of nutritional yeast when serving, to add a cheesy flavor.

PER SERVING (1 bowl or jar)

Calories: 396; Total Fat: 34g; Protein: 17g; Total Carbs: 5.5g; Fiber: 2.5g; Net Carbs: 3g

BUFFALO CHICKEN SALAD

SERVES 6 | PREP TIME: 10 MINUTES | COOK TIME: 20 MINUTES

EGG-FREE · NUT-FREE · PALEO/DAIRY-FREE OPTION · BULK PREP · UNDER 30 MINUTES

This is one of my go-to meal preps for lunch or dinner during the week. I make a big batch of buffalo chicken and use it in various meals like omelets, salads, and keto pizzas. You can even turn this into a 5-minute prep by replacing the chicken thighs with shredded, precooked rotisserie chicken.

FOR THE BUFFALO CHICKEN

1 cup hot sauce (I use Frank's RedHot Sauce)

1 tablespoon garlic powder

1 pound boneless, skinless chicken thighs

2 tablespoons butter, cubed

FOR THE SALAD

12 cups chopped romaine lettuce or spinach

6 ounces blue cheese or feta, crumbled

6 tablespoons ranch dressing

TO MAKE THE BUFFALO CHICKEN

1. Preheat the oven to 350°F.

2. In a glass baking dish, whisk together the hot sauce and garlic powder. Add the chicken and coat with the sauce. Top with the butter and bake for 15 to 20 minutes until the chicken is cooked through.

3. Let cool and then shred with a fork.

4. Store a few portions of the buffalo chicken in the refrigerator for an easy lunch or dinner during the week, and freeze the remaining portions.

TO MAKE ONE SERVING OF SALAD

Combine 2 cups of lettuce or spinach, 1 ounce of cheese, and 1 tablespoon of dressing. Top with 1 portion of chicken.

VARIATION TIP: Substitute feta (or any other cheese you like) for the blue cheese. Add a few slices of avocado in place of the lettuce.

MAKE IT PALEO/DAIRY-FREE: Leave out the cheese and instead sprinkle 1 tablespoon of nutritional yeast on top.

PER SERVING (1 salad)

Calories: 407; Total Fat: 31g; Protein: 26g; Total Carbs: 6g; Fiber: 2g; Net Carbs: 4g

GREEK SALAD IN A JAR

SERVES 4 | PREP TIME: 10 MINUTES | COOK TIME: 10 MINUTES

EGG-FREE · NUT-FREE · BULK PREP · UNDER 30 MINUTES

If you're looking to throw together a simple, grab-and-go lunch for the week, this is it. The mason jars make this salad easy to store and travel with. Don't worry about an extra container for the dressing, because it's layered in the jar so the dressing is only touching the ingredients that aren't prone to getting soggy.

8 bacon slices

8 tablespoons Fat-Burning Dressing (page 238)

8 cherry tomatoes, halved

2 cucumbers, diced (about 2 cups)

16 large olives, pitted and halved

1 cup crumbled feta cheese

4 cups chopped romaine lettuce

1. In a large skillet, cook the bacon over medium-high heat until crisp, 5 to 7 minutes. Remove to a paper towel and let cool.

2. In 4 quart-size, wide-mouth mason jars, divide and layer ingredients. Add to each jar in the following order: 2 tablespoons of dressing, 4 tomato halves, ½ cup cucumbers, 8 olive halves, ¼ cup feta cheese, 1 cup of romaine, and top with 2 crumbled bacon slices.

3. Secure the lids tightly and store in the refrigerator.

4. When ready to eat, shake well and pour into a bowl or eat it right out of the jar.

VARIATION TIP: Replace the crumbled bacon with shredded chicken, salami, or other meat of choice, and feel free to swap feta for your preferred cheese.

INGREDIENT TIP: If you're not in the mood to make the dressing, you can use oil and vinegar or your favorite sugar-free dressing.

PER SERVING (1 jar without dressing)

Calories: 224; Total Fat: 16g; Protein: 13g; Total Carbs: 7g; Fiber: 2.5g; Net Carbs: 4.5g

PER SERVING (1 jar with Fat-Burning Dressing)

Calories: 325; Total Fat: 27g; Protein: 13g; Total Carbs: 7.5g; Fiber: 2.5g; Net Carbs: 5g

JALAPEÑO BACON EGG SALAD

SERVES 4 | PREP TIME: 10 MINUTES | COOK TIME: 20 MINUTES

NUT-FREE · PALEO/DAIRY-FREE · BULK PREP · UNDER 30 MINUTES

Egg salad is one of the easiest breakfast or lunch meals to have on hand for a busy week. The only time-consuming part is boiling the eggs and cooking the bacon, which can be done ahead of time. The jalapeño gives this egg salad a spicy, crunchy twist. Enjoy it alone or serve it on a bed of lettuce or in lettuce cups. You can also serve it with veggies or Keto Crackers (page 136) for an extra crunch.

8 eggs

1 teaspoon vinegar

6 bacon slices

3 tablespoons mayonnaise

1 jalapeño pepper, seeded and finely chopped

1 tablespoon chopped chives

1 tablespoon Everything Seasoning (page 236)

1 teaspoon paprika

Sea salt

Freshly ground black pepper

1. Place the eggs in a medium pot and add enough cold water to cover them. Add a splash of vinegar (this makes the eggs easier to peel) and bring to a boil. Once boiling, remove the pot from the heat, cover, and let stand for 10 minutes. Meanwhile, fill a large bowl with water and ice. When the eggs are done, transfer them to the ice bath for another 10 minutes. When cooled, peel and roughly chop the eggs.

2. Meanwhile, in a large skillet, cook the bacon over medium-high heat until crisp, 5 to 7 minutes. Remove the bacon to a paper towel, reserving the bacon grease in the pan.

3. In a large bowl, combine the chopped eggs, mayonnaise, jalapeño, chives, seasoning, and paprika and then crumble the bacon on top. Mix well and season with salt and pepper.

4. Divide evenly among four glass containers and store in the refrigerator for a ready-made meal.

VARIATION TIP: Not in the mood for eggs? Swap them out for diced chicken, tuna, or other protein.

INGREDIENT TIP: I invested in an electric egg cooker on Amazon that was only about $15 and well worth it. The eggs come out perfectly every time and are super easy to peel.

PER SERVING (about ¾ cup)

Calories: 303; Total Fat: 25g; Protein: 17g; Total Carbs: 2.5g; Fiber: 1.5g; Net Carbs: 1g

CREAMY CHICKEN VEGETABLE SOUP

SERVES 8 | PREP TIME: 25 MINUTES | COOK TIME: 1 HOUR AND 45 MINUTES

NUT-FREE · PALEO/DAIRY-FREE OPTION · BULK PREP

I must admit, I've never been a big fan of soup for my main meal. However, this creamy chicken vegetable soup is on a whole other level. The flavor combination and richness of the broth combined with the hearty chunks of chicken and gooey melted cheese is so comforting and extremely filling. I make a big batch and store it in individual containers in the freezer for an easy lunch or dinner.

¼ cup butter or ghee

¼ medium onion, finely chopped (about ½ cup)

3 celery stalks, finely chopped

3 garlic cloves, minced

2 tablespoons Mediterranean Spice Blend (page 237) or Italian seasoning

1 jalapeño pepper, finely chopped

2 medium zucchini, chopped

4 cups Bone Broth (page 240)

¼ cup freshly squeezed lemon juice

8 ounces cream cheese, cut into pieces

1 cup grated Parmesan cheese

1 pound shredded rotisserie chicken

Sea salt

Freshly ground black pepper

1. In a large pot over medium heat, melt the butter or ghee. Add the onion, celery, garlic, and seasoning and sauté for 5 minutes. Add the jalapeño and zucchini and sauté for 10 minutes more.

2. Stir in the bone broth and bring to a boil. Reduce the heat to low and simmer for 45 minutes to 1 hour.

3. Add the lemon juice, cream cheese, Parmesan, and shredded chicken. Simmer for another 30 minutes. Season with salt and pepper.

4. To store, divide the soup into large glass jars (2 servings per jar) and freeze for easy meals throughout the coming weeks and months. Make sure to only fill the jars three-quarters full because the liquid will expand in the freezer.

MAKE IT PALEO/DAIRY-FREE: Replace the cream cheese and Parmesan with canned full-fat coconut milk.

PER SERVING (about 2 cups)

Calories: 336; Total Fat: 24g; Protein: 23g; Total Carbs: 7g; Fiber: 1.5g; Net Carbs: 5.5g

MEATBALL AND KALE PARMESAN SOUP

SERVES 8 | PREP TIME: 15 MINUTES | COOK TIME: 45 MINUTES

EGG-FREE · NUT-FREE · BULK PREP

This hearty soup brings in the antioxidant power of superfood kale, while spicing it up with some freshly made, spiced pork meatballs. Or, if you're pressed for time, you can substitute loose Italian sausage. Just be sure to check for fillers that include extra carbs.

2 pounds ground pork

½ teaspoon sea salt

1 teaspoon dried sage

1 teaspoon dried thyme

½ teaspoon ground allspice

8 cups Bone Broth (page 240)

1 medium yellow onion, diced

2 teaspoons Italian seasoning

½ teaspoon freshly squeezed lemon juice

2 teaspoons chopped fresh rosemary

3 garlic cloves, minced

2 bay leaves

1 cup grated Parmesan cheese

¾ cup heavy (whipping) cream

2 cups torn kale leaves

⅔ cup dry white wine

Sea salt

Freshly ground black pepper

Red pepper flakes, for garnish

1. In a large bowl, stir together the pork, salt, sage, thyme, and allspice until well combined. Form the mixture into ½-inch balls.

2. In a large stockpot, combine the bone broth, onion, Italian seasoning, lemon juice, rosemary, garlic, and bay leaves. Bring to a boil over medium-high heat. Reduce the heat to medium-low and let simmer, uncovered, for about 30 minutes.

3. Strain the solids from the broth, and return the broth to the stockpot.

4. Add the Parmesan and cream and cook, stirring, over low heat for about 5 minutes. Add the kale, wine, and meatballs. Cook for another 10 minutes or until the kale is tender. Taste and season with salt and pepper.

5. To serve, divide the soup among eight serving bowls and garnish with red pepper flakes. Store leftovers in airtight containers in the refrigerator for up to 4 days or in the freezer for up to 3 months.

PER SERVING (about 1½ cups)

Calories: 429; Total Fat: 33g; Protein: 28g; Total Carbs: 5g; Fiber: 1g; Net Carbs: 4g

BROCCOLI CHEDDAR PANCETTA SOUP

SERVES 6 | PREP TIME: 15 MINUTES | COOK TIME: 30 MINUTES

EGG-FREE · NUT-FREE · VEGETARIAN OPTION · BULK PREP

This hearty broccoli Cheddar soup blows Panera's broccoli cheese soup out the window any day. Plus, it's way lower in carbs and even creamier. One serving of this soup is super rich and fills you up fast. It gets thicker and more flavorful as it sits in the refrigerator overnight, so be sure to save some leftovers. Skip the baguette and serve with a few Keto Crackers (page 136).

2 ounces pancetta, diced

2 tablespoons butter or ghee

¼ medium onion, finely chopped (about ½ cup)

3 garlic cloves, minced

3 cups Bone Broth (page 240)

½ cup heavy (whipping) cream

2 cups broccoli florets, chopped into bite-size pieces

1 teaspoon garlic powder

1 teaspoon onion powder

1 teaspoon paprika

1 teaspoon salt

½ teaspoon freshly ground black pepper

Pinch cayenne pepper

½ tablespoon gelatin (or ½ teaspoon xanthan or guar gum), for thickening

2 cups shredded sharp Cheddar cheese

1. In a large pot over medium heat, cook the pancetta, stirring often, until crisp. Remove the pancetta pieces to a paper towel using a slotted spoon, leaving as much grease as possible in the pot.

2. Add the butter, onion, and garlic to the pot and sauté for 5 minutes.

3. Add the bone broth, cream, broccoli, garlic, onion, paprika, salt, pepper, and cayenne to the pot and stir well. Sprinkle in the gelatin and stir until well incorporated. Bring to a boil.

4. Once boiling, reduce the heat to low and simmer for 10 to 15 minutes, stirring occasionally.

5. Then, with the heat on low, gradually add the cheese, ½ cup at a time, stirring constantly. Once all of the cheese has been added, remove the pot from the heat. Sprinkle the pancetta pieces over the top and serve.

6. To store, divide the soup into glass jars and freeze for easy meals throughout the coming weeks and months. Make sure to only fill the jars three-quarters full because the liquid will expand as it freezes.

INGREDIENT TIP: Pancetta is an Italian-style bacon and is usually sold pre-diced or in slices in the deli section. Feel free to replace the pancetta with a few slices of bacon.

MAKE IT VEGETARIAN: Leave out the pancetta and add an extra tablespoon of butter or ghee. Replace the bone broth with vegetable broth.

PER SERVING (about 1½ cups)

Calories: 311; Total Fat: 29g; Protein: 17g; Total Carbs: 5.5g; Fiber: 1g; Net Carbs: 4.5g

KETO PHO WITH SHIRATAKI NOODLES

MAKES 4 BOWLS | PREP TIME: 20 MINUTES | COOK TIME: 10 MINUTES

EGG-FREE · NUT-FREE · PALEO/DAIRY-FREE · UNDER 30 MINUTES

Pho is actually an easy dish to make keto by swapping out the traditional noodles for shirataki noodles. Shirataki noodles, also called "miracle noodles," are made from the Japanese konjac plant and are practically carb- and calorie-free because they're made up of 97 percent water and 3 percent soluble fiber, called glucomannan. They're an amazing keto-friendly alternative and are extremely filling. The glucomannan does have a distinct scent, but it is easily washed away by rinsing them thoroughly before adding to your dish.

8 ounces sirloin, very thinly sliced

3 tablespoons coconut oil (or butter or ghee)

2 garlic cloves, minced

2 tablespoons liquid or coconut aminos

2 tablespoons fish sauce

1 teaspoon freshly grated or ground ginger

8 cups Bone Broth (page 240)

4 (7-ounce) packages shirataki noodles, drained and rinsed

1 cup bean sprouts

1 scallion, chopped

1 tablespoon toasted sesame seeds (optional)

1. Put the sirloin in the freezer while you prepare the broth and other ingredients (about 15 to 20 minutes). This makes it easier to slice.

2. In a large pot over medium heat, melt the coconut oil. Add the garlic and cook for 3 minutes. Then add the aminos, fish sauce, ginger, and bone broth. Bring to a boil.

3. Remove the beef from the freezer and slice it very thin.

4. Divide the noodles, beef, and bean sprouts evenly among four serving bowls. Carefully ladle 2 cups of broth into each bowl. Cover the bowls with plates and let sit for 3 to 5 minutes to cook the meat.

5. Serve garnished with the chopped scallion and sesame seeds (if using).

VARIATION TIP: Feel free to change up the vegetables and condiments to add more variety. Some examples include sliced jalapeños, chili sauce, baby bok choy, kale, soft-boiled egg, basil, cilantro, or mint.

PER SERVING (1 bowl)

Calories: 385; Total Fat: 29g; Protein: 23g; Total Carbs: 8g; Fiber: 3.5g; Net Carbs: 4.5g

MEATY KETO CHILI

SERVES 8 | PREP TIME: 15 MINUTES | COOK TIME: 50 MINUTES

EGG-FREE · NUT-FREE · PALEO/DAIRY-FREE · BULK PREP

It's hard to go wrong when it comes to chili, especially when there's bacon involved. This meaty chili is simple, flavorful, and a great option for lunch or dinner. Add your favorite keto-friendly toppings: sour cream, shredded cheese, jalapeños, or chopped scallions.

6 bacon slices

1 yellow onion, chopped

4 garlic cloves, minced

2 green chile peppers, finely chopped (or 1 [4-ounce] can green chilies)

2 tablespoons Mexican Spice Blend (page 237)

2 pounds ground beef

3 cups Bone Broth (page 240)

2 tablespoons tomato paste

1 teaspoon sea salt

½ teaspoon pepper

1 tablespoon gelatin (or ½ to 1 teaspoon xanthan or guar gum), for thickening

1. In a large skillet over medium heat, cook the bacon until crisp. Remove the bacon to a paper towel, leaving the fat in the skillet.

2. Add the onion, garlic, chiles, and Mexican spice blend to the skillet and cook, stirring frequently, for 5 minutes.

3. Add the ground beef to the pan and cook, stirring frequently, for about 5 more minutes until the meat is browned.

4. Pour the bone broth into the skillet and mix well. Add the tomato paste, salt, and pepper and sprinkle in the gelatin. Stir and bring to a boil.

5. Once boiling, reduce the heat to low and simmer for 30 minutes, stirring occasionally.

6. Crumble the bacon into the skillet and stir to combine.

7. Serve immediately or store in the refrigerator for up to 1 week or in the freezer for up to 2 months.

INGREDIENT TIP: Gelatin is a great alternative to cornstarch for thickening sauces. It's important to use a good quality gelatin so you get the numerous health benefits, like protecting your bones and joints, improving skin and gut health, and much more. I recommend the unflavored, grass-fed and pasture-raised beef gelatin from Aspen Naturals, Vital Proteins, or Great Lakes (these can be purchased online).

PER SERVING (about 1¼ cups)

Calories: 417; Total Fat: 33g; Protein: 25g; Total Carbs: 5g; Fiber: 1g; Net Carbs: 4g

BEEF SLOW COOKER STEW

SERVES 4 | PREP TIME: 15 MINUTES | COOK TIME: 10 HOURS ON LOW

EGG-FREE · NUT-FREE · PALEO/DAIRY-FREE

This stew, both meaty and brothy, will capture your heart, especially on cold winter nights. The radishes and carrot are added at the end so they retain some freshness in the stew when served right away.

2 tablespoons coconut oil or lard

1 pound beef chuck roast or pot roast, trimmed and cut into 2-inch cubes

1 shallot, chopped

2 garlic cloves, roughly chopped

4 cups Bone Broth (page 240), plus additional if needed

1 tablespoon balsamic vinegar

2 tablespoons tomato paste

2 tablespoons butter or ghee

1 large bay leaf

2 teaspoons dried thyme

1 teaspoon fresh winter savory

1 teaspoon sea salt

½ teaspoon freshly ground black pepper

2 cups cubed radishes

1 large carrot, sliced

1. Turn the slow cooker on and set it to low.

2. In a large skillet, heat the oil over medium-high heat. Add the beef and cook, without stirring, until browned on all sides, about 1 to 2 minutes per side. Remove the skillet from the heat.

3. In the slow cooker, combine the beef, shallot, garlic, bone broth, vinegar, tomato paste, butter, bay leaf, thyme, savory, salt, and pepper. Add additional broth if necessary to just cover the ingredients.

4. Cook on low for 9 to 10 hours, or on high for 6 to 7 hours.

5. About 2 hours before serving, add the radishes and carrot. Remove the bay leaf and season with salt..

6. To serve, divide the stew among four serving bowls. Store leftovers in airtight containers in the refrigerator for up to 6 days or in the freezer for up to 2 months.

RECIPE TIP: If you don't have a slow cooker, you can use a large Dutch oven or oven-safe pot and cook the stew for 4 to 6 hours at 300°F.

PER SERVING

Calories: 377; Total Fat: 25g; Protein: 29g; Total Carbs: 9g; Fiber: 2g; Net Carbs: 7g

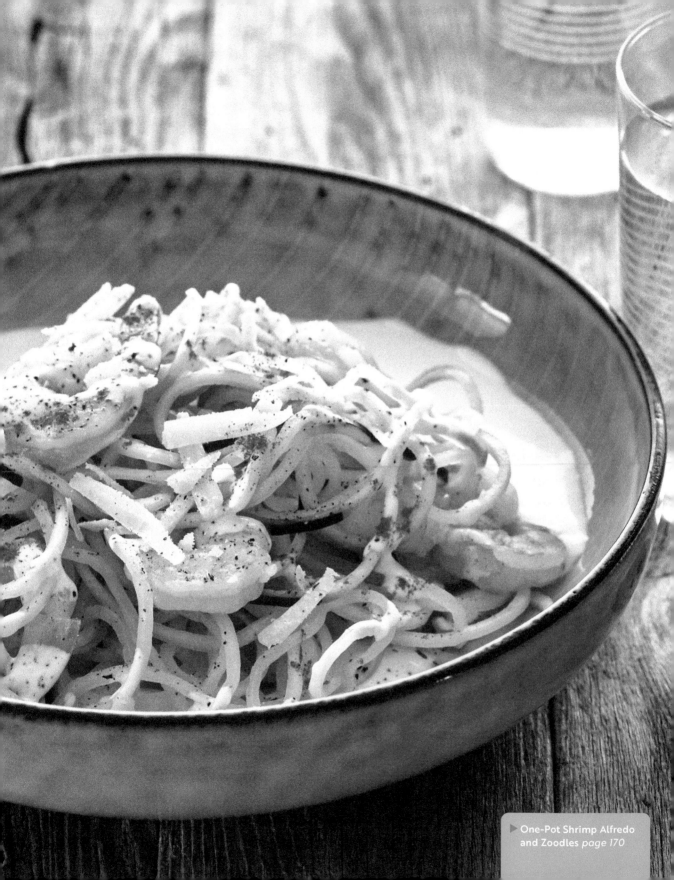

One-Pot Shrimp Alfredo and Zoodles *page 170*

Fish and Seafood

TUNA EGG SALAD

SERVES 4 | PREP TIME: 10 MINUTES

NUT-FREE · PALEO/DAIRY-FREE · BULK PREP · UNDER 30 MINUTES

I was a sucker for tuna sandwiches and melts growing up. There was a diner across the street from my apartment building in Manhattan that made the best tuna melts ever! The diner is still there to this day and I always indulge when I'm back home. They give me weird looks when I ask for it open-faced without the bread, but oh well, it's still delicious. This is my take on a tasty tuna salad that can be served with a few Keto Crackers (page 136), in lettuce cups, or even topped with a slice of cheese and melted until bubbly.

2 (5-ounce) cans tuna packed in water, drained

4 hard-boiled eggs, chopped

⅓ cup mayonnaise

2 tablespoons hulled sunflower seeds

2 teaspoons Dijon mustard

1 tablespoon Everything Seasoning (page 236)

¼ teaspoon sea salt

Pinch freshly ground black pepper

Pinch cayenne pepper (optional)

Fresh parsley, chopped, for garnish (optional)

1. In a medium bowl, combine the tuna, eggs, mayonnaise, sunflower seeds, mustard, and seasoning. Mix until well combined. Season with the salt and pepper and add the cayenne (if using).

2. Divide the tuna mixture evenly among four glass containers and store in the refrigerator for an easy, ready-made meal. Sprinkle with parsley before serving.

INGREDIENT TIP: Choose wild-caught tuna and make sure to use mayonnaise that's made with healthy oils such as avocado or olive oil. I like the Wild Planet brand for tuna and the Primal Kitchen or Chosen Foods brands for mayonnaise. Or you could make the mayonnaise from scratch.

VARIATION TIP: Not a fan of tuna? Swap it out for chicken, salmon, or another protein source.

PER SERVING (about 1 cup)

Calories: 351; Total Fat: 27g; Protein: 25g; Total Carbs: 2g; Fiber: 1g; Net Carbs: 1g

SIMPLE NUT-CRUSTED MAHI MAHI

SERVES 4 | PREP TIME: 5 MINUTES | COOK TIME: 15 MINUTES

PALEO/DAIRY-FREE · UNDER 30 MINUTES

A deliciously crunchy crust tops tender, flaky mahi mahi fillets in this simple recipe. Serve with roasted asparagus or sautéed spinach and you've got a quick, flavorful, and satisfying meal.

Coconut oil, for greasing

4 (4-ounce) mahi mahi fillets, rinsed and patted dry

1 teaspoon sea salt, plus a pinch

½ teaspoon freshly ground black pepper, plus a pinch

½ cup roasted and salted macadamia nuts, coarsely chopped

2 tablespoons almond flour (or crushed pork rinds)

½ teaspoon garlic powder

½ teaspoon onion powder

4 tablespoons mayonnaise

1. Preheat the oven to 400°F. Grease an 8-inch square baking dish with coconut oil.

2. Place the mahi mahi in the prepared baking dish.

3. Sprinkle each fillet with salt and pepper on both sides.

4. In small bowl, mix together the macadamia nuts, almond flour, garlic powder, onion powder, and a pinch salt and pepper.

5. Spread 1 tablespoon of mayonnaise on each fillet. Divide the nut mixture among the tops of the 4 fillets, gently patting it down so it adheres to the mayonnaise.

6. Bake for about 15 minutes until golden brown and cooked through.

VARIATION TIP: Swap cod, or any other fish you like, for the mahi mahi. You can also mix up the nuts and use pili nuts, pecans, walnuts, or another low-carb nut of choice.

INGREDIENT TIP: I use the Primal Kitchen or Chosen Foods brand of mayonnaise because they are made with avocado oil. You could also make your own home-made mayo.

PER SERVING (1 fillet)

Calories: 364; Total Fat: 28g; Protein: 24g; Total Carbs: 4g; Fiber: 2g; Net Carbs: 2g

SWEET AND SPICY OVEN-BAKED SALMON

SERVES 4 | PREP TIME: 10 MINUTES | COOK TIME: 20 MINUTES

EGG-FREE · NUT-FREE · PALEO/DAIRY-FREE · UNDER 30 MINUTES

Salmon is a super keto food because it's packed with healthy omega-3 fats and is a great source of protein. Make sure to avoid farm-raised salmon, which can contain added hormones, antibiotics, and other toxins, and opt for sustainable, wild-caught instead. This salmon recipe will light up your taste buds with the perfect combination of sweet and spicy. Serve with Garlic Butter Baby Bok Choy (page 226) for a quick, tasty meal.

1 pound salmon, rinsed and patted dry

1 serving Sweet and Spicy Sauce
(page 144)

1. Preheat the oven to 350°F. Line a baking sheet with aluminum foil.

2. Place the salmon, skin-side down, on the prepared baking sheet and fold up all four sides of the foil. Spoon the sauce over the salmon and then fold the sides of the foil over the salmon, covering it completely and sealing the foil closed.

3. Bake for 15 to 20 minutes until cooked through.

4. Cut into four equal portions and serve.

VARIATION TIP: Not in the mood for sweet and spicy? Switch it up and use the Garlic and Parmesan Sauce (page 143) instead.

INGREDIENT TIP: Choose wild-caught salmon over farm-raised to avoid added hormones, antibiotics, and other toxins.

PER SERVING
(1 [4-ounce] fillet with sauce)

Calories: 314; Total Fat: 22g; Protein: 26g; Total Carbs: 3g; Fiber: 0.3g; Net Carbs: 2.7g

SALMON-STUFFED PORTABELLA MUSHROOMS

SERVES 4 | PREP TIME: 5 MINUTES | COOK TIME: 25 MINUTES

NUT-FREE · PALEO/DAIRY-FREE OPTION · UNDER 30 MINUTES

Although not a very traditional combo, this recipe is surprisingly tasty. You can use canned or fresh salmon, as long as it is wild and sustainably caught. When buying canned salmon, look for skinless and boneless on the label. Wild Planet is the brand I use and it can be found in most grocery stores or online.

4 portabella mushroom caps

2 (6-ounce) cans wild-caught salmon (or freshly cooked wild-caught salmon)

4 ounces cream cheese, at room temperature

¼ cup mayonnaise

2 scallions, chopped

½ teaspoon paprika

½ teaspoon garlic powder

½ teaspoon sea salt

¼ teaspoon freshly ground black pepper

1 cup freshly grated Parmesan cheese

1. Preheat the oven to 350°F and line a baking sheet with parchment paper.

2. Clean the mushrooms, remove the stems, and carefully scrape the gills away with a spoon. Place them top down on the baking sheet.

3. In a large bowl, combine the salmon, cream cheese, mayonnaise, scallions, paprika, garlic powder, salt, and pepper. Mix well to combine.

4. Spoon the salmon mixture into the mushroom caps, dividing equally.

5. Sprinkle with the Parmesan and bake for 20 to 25 minutes until the mushrooms are tender and the cheese is bubbly.

VARIATION TIP: Make this a party appetizer by using small baby bella mushrooms instead of the large portabella mushrooms.

MAKE IT PALEO/DAIRY-FREE: Replace the cream cheese with another ¼ cup of mayonnaise and swap the Parmesan for a few tablespoons of nutritional yeast.

PER SERVING (1 mushroom cap)

Calories: 385; Total Fat: 29g; Protein: 26g; Total Carbs: 5g; Fiber: 1g; Net Carbs: 4g

HALIBUT IN A BUTTER AND GARLIC BLANKET

SERVES 4 | PREP TIME: 10 MINUTES | COOK TIME: 20 MINUTES

EGG-FREE · NUT-FREE · UNDER 30 MINUTES

This is a fantastic way to bake any type of white fish. The halibut in this recipe, a very mild fish, absorbs more than its fair share of butter, and since it's steamed in a little homemade foil pouch, even the steam seems to be made of butter. The pouch also keeps the fish moist.

Coconut oil, for greasing

4 (4-ounce) halibut fillets,
  about 1-inch thick

½ cup (1 stick) butter, cut into squares

2 tablespoons finely chopped scallion

1 tablespoon minced garlic

½ lemon

Sea salt

Freshly ground black pepper

1. Preheat the oven to 400°F.

2. Cut out four 12-inch squares of aluminum foil, and grease them with coconut oil. Place one halibut fillet on each foil square. Place two pats of butter on each fillet. Sprinkle the scallion and garlic over the fillets, dividing equally, and then squeeze the lemon half over the fillets, finally topping with a healthy sprinkle of salt and pepper.

3. Pull the sides of each foil square up to create a pouch around the halibut, and then roll the top like a paper lunch bag. The fish should be completely enclosed, but there should be room in the foil pouches to allow steam to circulate and cook the fish. Place the foil pouches on a large baking sheet.

4. Bake for about 20 minutes until the fish is opaque throughout.

5. Remove the fish from the foil pouches before serving but **save the "juice"** to serve over any veggies that you choose to serve with the dish.

VARIATION TIP: This method works great for any white fish, and even with chicken!

PER SERVING (1 fillet)

Calories: 313; Total Fat: 25g; Protein: 21g; Total Carbs: 1g; Fiber: 0g; Net Carbs: 1g

OMEGA-3 PIZZA

SERVES 2 | PREP TIME: 5 MINUTES | COOK TIME: 20 MINUTES

NUT-FREE · PALEO/DAIRY-FREE OPTION · UNDER 30 MINUTES

My good friends Robert Sikes and Crystal Love from the Keto Savage Kitchen inspired this recipe. Robert and Crystal came up with the idea of making a pizza crust out of mackerel, a nutrient-dense fish that is high in omega-3 fatty acids (something all of us need more of in our diets). I use the Wild Planet brand boneless and skinless mackerel fillets in extra-virgin olive oil for this recipe. It's similar to canned tuna, but even tastier in my opinion. Add whatever toppings you like (keto-friendly of course) and enjoy this completely guilt-free pizza.

2 (4.4-ounce) cans mackerel fillets, drained

¾ cup freshly grated Parmesan cheese, divided

1 egg

½ teaspoon garlic powder

½ teaspoon onion powder

½ teaspoon lemon-pepper seasoning (optional)

½ teaspoon sea salt

⅛ teaspoon freshly ground black pepper

2 tablespoons Easy Peasy Garlicky Pesto (page 245)

1. Preheat the oven to 400°F. Line a baking sheet or pizza pan with parchment paper.

2. In a large bowl, break up the drained mackerel into small pieces with a fork. Add ¼ cup of Parmesan, the egg, garlic powder, onion powder, lemon-pepper seasoning (if using), salt, and pepper and mix until well combined. Pour the mixture onto the baking sheet. Place another piece of parchment paper over the mixture and form it into a crust, making sure to pack it down tightly, spreading the mixture into a thin, even layer.

3. Remove the parchment paper from the top and bake for about 15 minutes until golden brown.

4. Add the pesto and the remaining ½ cup of Parmesan and bake or broil for another 3 to 4 minutes until the cheese is melted.

MAKE IT PALEO/DAIRY-FREE: Replace the cheese with nutritional yeast or pork rinds and your preferred toppings.

PER SERVING (½ crust)

Calories: 284; Total Fat: 18g; Protein: 29g; Total Carbs: 1.5g; Fiber: 0g; Net Carbs: 1.5g

PER SERVING (½ crust with toppings)

Calories: 431; Total Fat: 31g; Protein: 35g; Total Carbs: 3g; Fiber: 0.5g; Net Carbs: 2.5g

CRISPY FISH STICKS WITH TARTAR SAUCE

SERVES 4 | PREP TIME: 10 MINUTES | COOK TIME: 15 MINUTES

NUT-FREE · PALEO/DAIRY-FREE OPTION · UNDER 30 MINUTES

The coating for these fish sticks is probably not what you're used to, but I promise you won't even be able to tell the difference once you crunch into these bad boys. The key is to opt for high-quality pork rinds that smell and taste great. I like the Bacon's Heir or EPIC brands. They even sell them already crushed as "Pork Panko," or you can get the whole ones and use a coffee/spice grinder or food processor to crush them.

FOR THE FISH STICKS

Avocado or coconut oil, for greasing

1 egg, lightly beaten

1 scoop unflavored MCT powder
   (or collagen powder)

Pinch sea salt

Pinch freshly ground black pepper

1 cup freshly grated Parmesan cheese

½ cup crushed pork rinds

1 teaspoon garlic powder

1 teaspoon onion powder

1 teaspoon paprika

1 pound cod fillets, rinsed, patted dry,
   and cut into 1-by-4-inch pieces

FOR THE SAUCE

4 tablespoons mayonnaise

1 pickle spear, finely chopped

1 teaspoon freshly squeezed
   lemon juice

½ teaspoon onion powder

½ teaspoon garlic powder

Pinch sea salt

Pinch freshly ground black pepper

1 teaspoon chopped fresh dill
   (optional)

Dash low-carb sweetener (optional)

TO MAKE THE FISH STICKS

1. Preheat the oven to 400°F. Line a rimmed baking sheet with aluminum foil. Place a wire rack over the baking sheet and lightly grease the rack with oil.

2. Put the lightly beaten egg in a shallow bowl. In another shallow bowl, combine the MCT powder, salt, and pepper.

3. In a third bowl, combine the Parmesan, pork rinds, garlic powder, onion powder, and paprika.

4. Dip the fish in the MCT mixture to coat both sides, shaking off the excess. Next, dip in the egg and then into the Parmesan mixture, patting to help the coating adhere. Place the fish on the wire rack.

5. Bake for 12 to 15 minutes until golden brown.

TO MAKE THE SAUCE

1. In a small bowl, mix together the mayonnaise, chopped pickle, lemon juice, onion powder, and garlic powder. Add the salt, pepper, dill (if using), and sweetener (if using).

2. Serve immediately or store in an airtight container in the refrigerator for up to 2 days.

MAKE IT PALEO/DAIRY-FREE: Replace the cheese with ¼ cup nutritional yeast.

INGREDIENT TIP: If you're not a fan of pork rinds, feel free to substitute with almond meal or more cheese.

PER SERVING (3 or 4 Fish Sticks)

Calories: 220; Total Fat: 10g; Protein: 31g; Total Carbs: 1.5g; Fiber: 0.5g; Net Carbs: 1g

PER SERVING (2 tablespoons Tartar Sauce)

Calories: 94; Total Fat: 10g; Protein: 0g; Total Carbs: 1g; Fiber: 0.3g; Net Carbs: 0.7g

PER SERVING (3 or 4 Fish Sticks + 2 tablespoons Tartar Sauce)

Calories: 314; Total Fat: 20g; Protein: 31g; Total Carbs: 2.5g; Fiber: 0.8g; Net Carbs: 1.7g

ONE-POT SHRIMP ALFREDO AND ZOODLES

SERVES 5 | PREP TIME: 10 MINUTES | COOK TIME: 25 MINUTES

EGG-FREE · NUT-FREE

Whoever came up with the idea of making noodles out of zucchini, also known as zoodles, is a genius! Zoodles have a fraction of the carbs and calories compared to regular spaghetti and they're a perfect replacement for practically any dish that calls for pasta. This one-pot shrimp Alfredo is rich, creamy, and kicks that comfort food craving in the butt!

FOR THE ZOODLES

3 medium zucchini (about 21 ounces
    or 600 grams if using
    pre-prepped zoodles)

1 teaspoon sea salt

FOR THE SHRIMP AND SAUCE

2 tablespoons butter or ghee

3 garlic cloves, minced

1 pound shrimp, peeled and deveined

4 ounces cream cheese,
    at room temperature

½ cup heavy (whipping) cream

½ teaspoon sea salt

¼ teaspoon freshly ground
    black pepper

1 cup freshly grated Parmesan cheese

¼ teaspoon cayenne pepper (optional)

TO MAKE THE ZOODLES

1. Trim off the ends of the zucchini. Using a vegetable spiral slicer, swirl the zucchini into noodle shapes (zoodles).

2. Lay the zoodles on a kitchen towel and sprinkle with the salt. Let sit while you prepare the Alfredo sauce.

3. While the sauce is simmering, fold the zoodles up in the towel and squeeze out as much water as you can.

TO MAKE THE SHRIMP AND SAUCE

1. In a large pot, melt the butter over medium heat. Add the garlic and cook for 3 minutes until fragrant. Add the shrimp and cook for 4 to 6 minutes, just until the shrimp start to turn pink. Remove the shrimp to a plate.

2. Add the cream cheese to the pot and whisk until melted. Pour in the cream slowly, whisking constantly. Add the salt and pepper. Let the sauce simmer for 5 to 10 minutes, whisking often, until thickened.

3. Remove the pot from the heat and stir in the Parmesan and cayenne (if using). Taste and adjust the salt and pepper to your liking.

4. Add the zoodles, cover, and cook for 5 minutes. The zoodles will release a bit of water, which will thin out the thick sauce a bit.

5. Add the shrimp and toss before serving.

RECIPE TIP: Prep the zoodles ahead of time and store them in the refrigerator in an airtight container for up to 1 week. Alternatively, most grocery stores now sell already prepped zoodles, although they're a little more costly than making them yourself.

PER SERVING

Calories: 329; Total Fat: 25g; Protein: 20g; Total Carbs: 6g; Fiber: 1g; Net Carbs: 5g

SHEET-PAN CAJUN CRAB LEGS AND VEGGIES

SERVES 6 | PREP TIME: 15 MIN | COOK TIME: 30 MINUTES

EGG-FREE · NUT-FREE · PALEO/DAIRY-FREE OPTION

Crab legs are not only carb-free, they're also packed with good fats, nutrients, and minerals. Dipped in melted butter with Cajun seasoning, they're pure savory heaven!

Coconut oil, for greasing

2 zucchini, halved lengthwise
  and sliced

3 cups roughly chopped cauliflower

10 tablespoons butter or ghee,
  melted, divided

2 tablespoons Cajun seasoning

1 tablespoon minced garlic

6 ounces Polish sausages or bratwurst,
  cut into rounds ½-inch thick

2 pounds frozen snow crab legs
  (about two clusters), thawed in the
  refrigerator overnight or for a few
  minutes under cold running water

½ lemon

Chopped fresh parsley, for garnish

1. Preheat the oven to 450°F. Line a large baking sheet with aluminum foil and grease the foil with oil.

2. Arrange the zucchini halves cut-side up on the prepared baking sheet. Add the cauliflower and spread it out in an even layer.

3. In a small bowl, stir together 5 tablespoons of melted butter, Cajun seasoning, and garlic until well mixed. Pour half of the butter mixture over the veggies, making sure to cover the cauliflower.

4. Bake for 15 to 20 minutes until the veggies are tender.

5. Place the sausage slices among the vegetables. Break up the crab legs and add them to the pan. Drizzle with the remaining butter mixture. Bake for an additional 10 minutes.

6. Squeeze the lemon half over the top, garnish with parsley, and serve immediately with the remaining 5 tablespoons of butter for dipping.

VARIATION TIP: Don't like crab? Substitute shrimp instead! Want to make it Paleo? Use ghee instead of butter.

PER SERVING

Calories: 415; Total Fat: 29g; Protein: 33g; Total Carbs: 5.5g; Fiber: 2g; Net Carbs: 3.5g

SHRIMP SCAMPI

SERVES 4 | PREP TIME: 5 MINUTES | COOK TIME: 10 MINUTES

EGG-FREE · NUT-FREE · UNDER 30 MINUTES

When it comes to finding quick and easy seafood recipes that don't require a ton of ingredients, this melt-in-your mouth shrimp scampi is a perfect choice. Serve it with a side of Zesty Roasted Broccoli (page 227) or on top of Zoodles (page 170).

4 tablespoons butter or ghee

4 garlic cloves, minced

½ cup Bone Broth (page 240)

½ teaspoon sea salt

¼ teaspoon freshly ground black pepper

2 pounds shrimp, peeled and deveined

¼ cup freshly squeezed lemon juice

Chopped fresh parsley, for garnish

1. In a large pan, melt the butter over medium heat. Add the garlic and cook for 3 minutes until fragrant.

2. Add the bone broth, salt, and pepper and bring to a simmer. Reduce the liquid by half (about 2 minutes).

3. Add the shrimp and cook for 4 to 6 minutes, just until the shrimp start to turn pink. Add the lemon juice. Sprinkle parsley over the shrimp to serve.

VARIATION TIP: You can swap the shrimp for another protein source such as chicken or halibut, or even remove the protein and use the buttery garlic sauce to top veggies for a quick, savory side dish.

PER SERVING

Calories: 253; Total Fat: 13g; Protein: 31g; Total Carbs: 3g; Fiber: 0g; Net Carbs: 3g

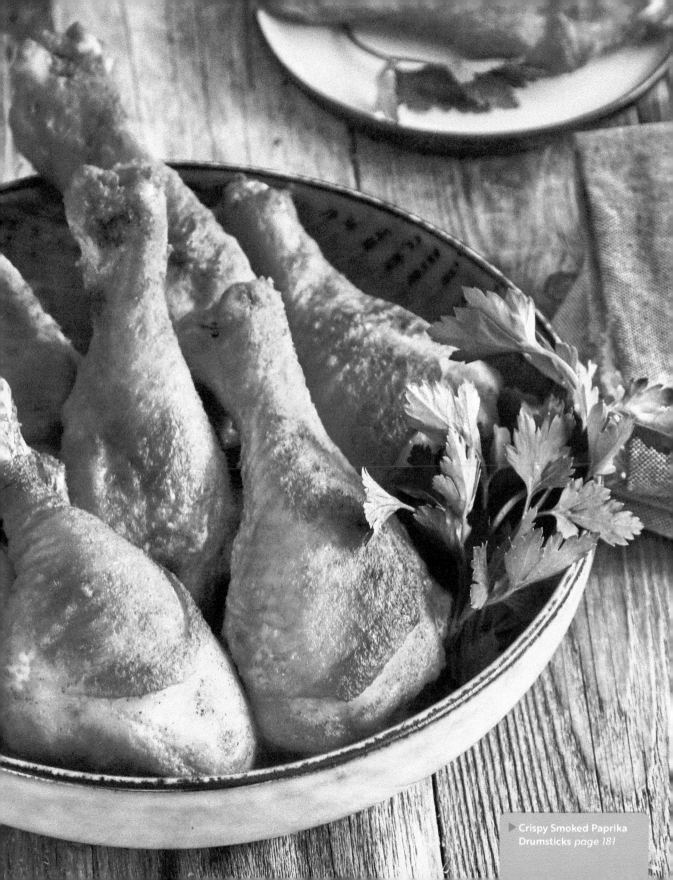

Crispy Smoked Paprika Drumsticks *page 181*

9

Poultry

HERBED CHICKEN SKEWERS

SERVES 4 | PREP TIME: 10 MINUTES PLUS 1 HOUR TO MARINATE | COOK TIME: 25 MINUTES

EGG-FREE · NUT-FREE · PALEO/DAIRY-FREE

These incredibly simple and savory chicken skewers are great for an easy weeknight dinner with some veggies, or as an appetizer at a barbecue. Either way, the Italian dressing locks into the meat and tenderizes it, making this a delicious meal option with a familiar flavor even the kids will love.

1 pound, boneless, skinless chicken breasts

1 cup Zesty Parmesan Italian Dressing (page 239)

1 teaspoon Italian seasoning

Freshly ground black pepper

1. Cut the chicken breasts into long thin strips, about 1 inch wide.

2. Combine the chicken, Italian dressing, and Italian seasoning in a resealable plastic bag and marinate in the refrigerator for at least 1 hour.

3. Soak 12 bamboo skewers in water for at least 10 minutes.

4. Preheat the oven or grill to 350°F.

5. Remove the chicken from the refrigerator and skewer it lengthwise for a total of 12 skewers.

6. If cooking on a grill, cook directly. If cooking in the oven, line and grease a baking sheet. Crack some fresh pepper over each of the skewers.

7. Place the skewers on the grill or in the oven for about 15 minutes, then flip and cook another 5 to 10 minutes or until cooked through.

RECIPE TIP: The longer you marinate, the more tender and flavorful the chicken will be. Don't forget to soak your skewers or they will burn in the grill or oven.

PER SERVING (3 skewers)

Calories: 288; Total Fat: 20g; Protein: 26g; Total Carbs: 1g; Fiber: 0g; Net Carbs: 1g

HARISSA COCONUT CHICKEN

SERVES 4 | PREP TIME: 5 MINUTES | COOK TIME: 20 MINUTES

EGG-FREE · NUT-FREE · UNDER 30 MINUTES

If you're looking for a super quick, extremely flavorful meal that can be prepared using only one pan, in about 20 minutes, look no further. This harissa coconut chicken is simple to make and delicious served over cauliflower rice, zoodles, or in lettuce wraps. Harissa paste is a spicy and aromatic chili paste that can be found in the international aisle of most grocery stores. If you can't find it, you can substitute regular chili paste.

2 tablespoons butter or ghee

1 pound boneless, skinless chicken thighs (or breast)

Sea salt

Freshly ground black pepper

½ cup unsweetened, full-fat canned coconut milk

2 tablespoons harissa paste

1. In a medium pan, melt the butter or ghee over medium heat.

2. Add the chicken and season with salt and pepper. Cook for 5 minutes and then flip and cook for another 5 minutes or until browned. Remove the chicken from the pan.

3. Add the coconut milk and harissa paste to the pan with the chicken drippings. Whisk the mixture together and bring to a boil. Return the chicken to the pan and simmer for about 10 minutes until cooked through.

INGREDIENT TIP: Not in the mood to cook chicken thighs? Grab a rotisserie chicken from the store, pull it off the bone, and add it to a pan with the coconut harissa sauce for a 5-minute meal.

PER SERVING

Calories: 381; Total Fat: 29g; Protein: 28g; Total Carbs: 2g; Fiber: 0g; Net Carbs: 2g

BUFFALO CHICKEN PIZZA

SERVES 6 | PREP TIME: 10 MINUTES | COOK TIME: 20 MINUTES

PALEO/DAIRY-FREE OPTION · UNDER 30 MINUTES

If you follow me on Instagram (@KillinItKeto), you know that this is my all-time favorite keto meal. I grew up eating New York–style pizza, so you know this has to be a winner if I'm recommending it. The crust is super easy to make and actually turns out like a real pizza crust (no fork and knife needed with this one). Not a fan of buffalo chicken? Substitute any of your favorite keto-friendly toppings like Alfredo, pesto, sugar-free barbecue sauce, or low-sugar tomato sauce and pepperoni, sausage, and whatever cheese you like.

1 batch Keto Dough (page 242, traditional, Paleo/dairy-free, or nut-free)

1½ teaspoons garlic powder, divided

½ teaspoon onion powder

½ teaspoon salt

½ cup hot sauce, such as Frank's RedHot Sauce

2 tablespoons butter, melted

2 cups shredded rotisserie chicken

½ cup shredded Cheddar cheese

1. Preheat the oven to 425°F. Line a pizza pan or baking sheet with parchment paper or a silicone mat.

2. Place the dough on the prepared baking sheet and top with another piece of parchment paper. Roll out the dough until it is about ¼- to ½-inch thick. Remove the top piece of parchment and sprinkle the dough evenly with ½ teaspoon of garlic powder and the onion powder and salt. Using a fork, poke holes all over the crust.

3. Bake for 12 to 15 minutes until golden brown.

4. While the crust is baking, make the topping. In a large bowl, whisk together the hot sauce, butter, and the remaining 1 teaspoon of garlic powder. Reserve 2 tablespoons of the sauce mixture for the crust and then add the shredded chicken to the mixture. Mix until the chicken is well coated.

5. Remove the crust from the oven and top with the reserved sauce, then the chicken mixture and cheese. Bake for another 3 to 5 minutes until the cheese is melted.

MAKE IT PALEO/DAIRY-FREE: Use the dairy-free keto dough and substitute the cheese for dairy-free cheese, or leave it out and use other suggested toppings.

INGREDIENT TIP: Make your own shredded chicken by simply baking chicken thighs or breasts in the oven for 20 to 25 minutes at 350°F and shred with a fork.

PER SERVING
(⅙ pizza using Traditional Keto Crust)

Calories: 350; Total Fat: 26g; Protein: 24g; Total Carbs: 5g; Fiber: 1.5g; Net Carbs: 3.5g

PER SERVING
(⅙ pizza using Paleo/Dairy-Free Keto Crust)

Calories: 363; Total Fat: 27g; Protein: 25g; Total Carbs: 5g; Fiber: 2g; Net Carbs: 3g

PER SERVING
(⅙ pizza using Nut-Free Keto Crust)

Calories: 288; Total Fat: 20g; Protein: 22g; Total Carbs: 5g; Fiber: 2g; Net Carbs: 3g

CRACKLING CREOLE CRISPY CHICKEN THIGHS

SERVES 4 | PREP TIME: 10 MINUTES | COOK TIME: 50 MINUTES

EGG-FREE · NUT-FREE · PALEO/DAIRY-FREE

For an easy-as-heck-weeknight dinner on a budget, these feisty chicken thighs can be thrown together easily and cooked up fast. Chicken thighs are some of the least expensive meats you can purchase, and the dark meat is slightly higher in fat than white meat while also being higher in iron, zinc, B vitamins, and other essential vitamins.

Coconut or olive oil, for greasing

¼ teaspoon paprika

¼ teaspoon onion powder

¼ teaspoon garlic powder

⅛ teaspoon dried oregano

⅛ teaspoon dried basil

⅛ teaspoon dried thyme

⅛ teaspoon dried rosemary

⅛ teaspoon dried parsley

⅛ teaspoon cayenne pepper

4 skin-on, bone-in chicken thighs

1 yellow onion, quartered

8 garlic cloves, peeled and left whole

¼ cup extra-virgin olive oil

1 tablespoon freshly squeezed lemon juice

1. Preheat the oven to 350°F. Grease a cast iron (or other oven-safe) skillet with oil.

2. In a large bowl, stir together the paprika, onion powder, garlic powder, oregano, basil, thyme, rosemary, parsley, and cayenne. Add the chicken and toss to coat. Place the chicken in the prepared skillet, skin-side up.

3. Separate the thighs with the quartered onion and then sprinkle the whole garlic cloves throughout the skillet, preferably so that they are touching the bottom.

4. Drizzle the oil over the chicken and then the lemon juice.

5. Bake in the oven for 30 to 40 minutes until cooked through and the juices run clear. Baste the breasts with juice from the bottom of the skillet.

6. Turn the oven to broil and broil for 5 to 10 minutes, watching closely, until the skin has crisped up to your liking.

7. Remove from the oven, break apart the onion, and enjoy the chicken with the onions and caramelized garlic cloves alongside your favorite vegetable.

PER SERVING (1 thigh)

Calories: 392; Total Fat: 32g; Protein: 20g; Total Carbs: 6g; Fiber: 1g; Net Carbs: 5g

CRISPY SMOKED PAPRIKA DRUMSTICKS

SERVES 6 | PREP TIME: 5 MINUTES | COOK TIME: 45 MINUTES

EGG-FREE · NUT-FREE · PALEO/DAIRY-FREE OPTION

This drumstick recipe is perfect for those hectic weeknights when you're looking for something easy with minimal cleanup. The smoked paprika and cayenne give these drumsticks a nice kick. I usually pair them with Bacon-Wrapped Asparagus Bundles (page 229) or Slow Cooker Creamed Spinach and Artichoke (page 233).

Oil or cooking spray, for greasing

1 tablespoon smoked paprika

1 tablespoon garlic powder

1 tablespoon onion powder

1 teaspoon baking powder

1 teaspoon sea salt

½ teaspoon freshly ground black pepper

¼ teaspoon cayenne pepper

2 tablespoons nutritional yeast (optional)

6 chicken drumsticks, patted dry

2 tablespoons butter, melted

1. Preheat the oven to 300°F. Line a baking sheet with aluminum foil and place a baking rack on top. Grease or spray the rack with oil to prevent the chicken from sticking.

2. In a paper or resealable plastic bag, combine the paprika, garlic powder, onion powder, baking powder, salt, pepper, cayenne, and nutritional yeast (if using), and shake well. Add the drumsticks to the bag and shake until they are well coated with the spice mixture.

3. Place the drumsticks on the prepared baking rack and cook for 25 minutes.

4. After 25 minutes, raise the oven heat to 400°F. Brush the drumsticks with the melted butter and cook for an additional 20 minutes or until crispy.

5. Remove from the oven and let cool for 5 minutes before serving.

MAKE IT PALEO/DAIRY-FREE: Use ghee if tolerated or replace with tallow or lard.

RECIPE TIP: To get the chicken thighs even crispier, set your oven to broil for the last 3 to 5 minutes of cooking.

PER SERVING (1 drumstick)

Calories: 200; Total Fat: 12g; Protein: 20g; Total Carbs: 3g; Fiber: 1g; Net Carbs: 2g

EASY MEXICAN CHICKEN CASSEROLE

SERVES 6 | PREP TIME: 10 MINUTES | COOK TIME: 30 MINUTES

EGG-FREE · NUT-FREE · BULK PREP

This quick and simple dish is packed with deliciousness, and the green chiles and chipotles add a spicy kick. If you're sensitive to spice, omit one or use less of each. If you're pressed for time, use a store-bought rotisserie chicken instead of cooking your own chicken thighs.

2 tablespoons butter, ghee, or coconut oil, plus more for greasing

1 pound skinless, boneless chicken thighs

Pinch sea salt

Pinch freshly ground black pepper

½ cup chopped onion

4 cups fresh or frozen riced cauliflower

4 tablespoons roasted and chopped canned or jarred green chiles

1 tablespoon Mexican Spice Blend (page 237)

½ cup sour cream

1 cup shredded pepper Jack cheese

1 cup shredded sharp Cheddar cheese, divided

2 tablespoons chopped chipotles in adobo sauce (optional)

1. Preheat the oven to 425°F. Grease a 9-by-13-inch baking dish with butter, ghee, or oil.

2. Place the chicken in the prepared baking dish and sprinkle with salt and pepper. Bake for 15 minutes or until cooked through.

3. While the chicken cooks, melt 2 tablespoons of butter or ghee or heat the oil in a large pan over medium heat. Add the onion, cauliflower, green chiles, and Mexican spice blend. Cook for 15 to 20 minutes, stirring occasionally, until the cauliflower is cooked through.

4. When the chicken is finished, remove it from the baking dish, let cool for 5 minutes, and then shred it using two forks. Pour out any excess liquid remaining in the casserole dish.

5. Add the shredded chicken to the cauliflower mixture along with the sour cream, pepper Jack, ½ cup of Cheddar, and chipotles. Mix well and pour into the baking dish. Top with the remaining ½ cup of Cheddar and bake for about 10 minutes until the cheese is melted and slightly browned.

6. Let cool for 5 minutes before serving.

PER SERVING (⅙ casserole)

Calories: 430; Total Fat: 30g; Protein: 31g; Total Carbs: 9g; Fiber: 3g; Net Carbs: 6g

QUICK KETO BUTTER CHICKEN

SERVES 4 | PREP TIME: 5 MINUTES | COOK TIME: 20 MINUTES

EGG-FREE · NUT-FREE · PALEO/DAIRY-FREE OPTION · UNDER 30 MINUTES

This is a quick and easy take on the classic butter chicken recipe. It's creamy, flavorful, and ready in no time. Serve it over cauliflower or shirataki rice for a filling dinner and enjoy the leftovers all week long as the flavors develop even more while it stores in the refrigerator.

1 pound boneless, skinless chicken thighs, cut into bite-size pieces

1½ tablespoons Indian Spice Blend (page 236)

2 tablespoons ghee or butter

½ cup chopped onion

½ cup heavy (whipping) cream

1 tablespoon tomato paste

½ teaspoon sea salt

¼ teaspoon freshly ground black pepper

1. In a large bowl, toss the chicken with the Indian spice blend until the chicken is well coated.

2. In a large skillet, melt the ghee over medium heat. Add the onion and cook for 3 minutes.

3. Raise the heat to medium-high and add the chicken. Cook for 5 to 7 minutes, stirring occasionally, until the chicken is browned all over. Reduce the heat to medium-low and stir in the cream, tomato paste, salt, and pepper. Let simmer for 10 to 15 minutes, stirring occasionally, until the sauce thickens.

MAKE IT PALEO/DAIRY-FREE: Replace the cream with unsweetened, full-fat canned coconut milk.

RECIPE TIP: Double or triple the recipe and freeze the leftovers for a yummy lunch or dinner later on.

PER SERVING

Calories: 323; Total Fat: 23g; Protein: 24g; Total Carbs: 5g; Fiber: 1g; Net Carbs: 4g

TURKEY POT PIE

SERVES 6 | PREP TIME: 10 MINUTES | COOK TIME: 45 MINUTES

EGG-FREE · NUT-FREE OPTION · PALEO/DAIRY-FREE OPTION

This recipe takes a little extra effort, but the final outcome will have your mouth watering for days. I use chopped broccoli florets and mushrooms instead of traditional pot pie veggies like carrots and peas because it helps keep the carb count in check (feel free to use other lower-carb veggies of your choice).

FOR THE FILLING

2 tablespoons butter, ghee, or coconut oil, plus more for greasing

½ cup chopped onion

3 garlic cloves, minced

2 cups chopped broccoli florets

2 cups sliced mushrooms

1 tablespoon Italian seasoning

1 teaspoon sea salt

½ teaspoon freshly ground black pepper

½ cup Bone Broth (page 240)

¼ cup heavy (whipping) cream

1 tablespoon gelatin (or ½ teaspoon xanthan or guar gum), for thickening

12 ounces precooked turkey (or chicken), chopped or shredded (about 2½ cups)

FOR THE CRUST

1 batch Keto Dough (page 242, traditional, Paleo/dairy-free, or nut-free, made with 2 teaspoons Italian seasoning)

TO MAKE THE FILLING

1. Preheat the oven to 400°F. Grease a 9-inch square baking dish with butter, ghee, or oil.

2. In a large pot, melt 2 tablespoons of butter or ghee over medium heat. Add the onion and garlic and cook for 3 minutes until fragrant. Add the broccoli, mushrooms, Italian seasoning, salt, and pepper. Cook for 5 minutes. Add the broth, cream, and gelatin. Stir and bring to a boil.

3. Once boiling, reduce the heat to medium-low and let simmer for 10 minutes, stirring occasionally, until the mixture thickens.

4. Add the turkey to the vegetable mixture and stir to combine. Pour the mixture into the prepared baking dish.

TO MAKE THE CRUST

1. Place the dough on a piece of parchment paper. Form the dough into a square and then place another piece of parchment paper over the dough. Roll out the dough until it is just slightly bigger than the baking dish. Remove the top piece of parchment.

2. Carefully flip the dough over the top of the filling in the baking dish, using a spatula to peel it away from the parchment paper if it sticks. Crimp the dough around the edges and make several slits in the top with a knife. Bake for 20 to 25 minutes until golden brown.

3. Let cool for 5 minutes and serve.

MAKE IT PALEO/DAIRY-FREE: Use dairy-free dough and replace the cream with unsweetened nut/seed milk (coconut, almond, hemp, cashew).

RECIPE TIP: You can make individual pot pies by evenly dividing the filling and dough between six 6-ounce ramekins.

PER SERVING (⅙ pie using Traditional Keto Dough)

Calories: 386; Total Fat: 26g; Protein: 30g; Total Carbs: 8g; Fiber: 3g; Net Carbs: 5g

PER SERVING
(⅙ pie using Paleo/Dairy-Free Keto Dough)

Calories: 405; Total Fat: 27g; Protein: 32g; Total Carbs: 8.5g; Fiber: 3.5g; Net Carbs: 5g

PER SERVING
(⅙ pie using Nut-Free Keto Dough)

Calories: 326; Total Fat: 20g; Protein: 28g; Total Carbs: 8.5g; Fiber: 3.5g; Net Carbs: 5g

SPINACH, MUSHROOM, AND FETA–STUFFED MEATLOAF

SERVES 6 | PREP TIME: 10 MINUTES | COOK TIME: 45 MINUTES

EGG-FREE · NUT-FREE · PALEO/DAIRY-FREE OPTION · BULK PREP

Stuffed meatloaf may sound complicated but it's actually pretty darn easy and adds a whole new flair to your typical meatloaf dish. I love the combination of spinach, mushrooms, and feta, but you can switch up the veggies and cheese as you like. The Mediterranean Spice Blend (page 237) gives this meatloaf a nice flavor, but I've also used Italian seasoning or sometimes just a mixture of spices that I have on hand. Use the spices you enjoy and make it your own!

2 tablespoons butter, ghee, or coconut oil, plus more for greasing

8 cups fresh spinach (or 8 ounces frozen)

¼ cup chopped onion

2 cups chopped mushrooms (about 6 ounces)

2 garlic cloves, minced

2 tablespoons Mediterranean Spice Blend (page 237), divided

1 teaspoon sea salt, divided

½ teaspoon freshly ground black pepper, divided

Pinch red pepper flakes

1½ pounds ground turkey or chicken

1 cup feta cheese, crumbled

2 tablespoons heavy (whipping) cream

½ teaspoon xanthan or guar gum

1. Preheat the oven to 375°F. Lightly grease an 8-by-4-inch loaf pan with butter, ghee, or coconut oil.

2. In a large microwave-safe bowl, cook the spinach in the microwave for 3 minutes if using fresh and 4 to 5 minutes if using frozen. If using frozen spinach, let cool for a few minutes after cooking then squeeze out excess liquid.

3. Meanwhile, in a medium skillet, melt the butter over medium heat. Add the onion, mushrooms, garlic, 1 tablespoon of Mediterranean spice blend, ½ teaspoon of salt, ¼ teaspoon of pepper, and the red pepper flakes. Cook for 5 to 7 minutes until the onion and mushrooms start to soften.

4. In a medium bowl, combine the ground turkey and the remaining 1 tablespoon of Mediterranean spice blend, ½ teaspoon of salt, and ¼ teaspoon of pepper. Mix until well combined.

5. Add the mushroom-onion mixture and feta cheese to the spinach and stir to mix well.

6. To assemble, put two-thirds of the meat in the prepared baking pan and push it up the sides to form a well in the middle. Add the spinach filling and smooth out the top. Top with the remaining meat mixture and spread it out to cover the entire filling.

7. Bake for 20 minutes and then carefully remove the pan from the oven and pour the excess juice into a small microwave-safe bowl. Return the meatloaf to the oven and cook for another 10 to 15 minutes until cooked through.

8. Meanwhile, whisk the cream and xanthan gum into the juice and then microwave for 1 to 2 minutes. Whisk until thickened to a gravy consistency.

9. When the meatloaf is cooked through, remove it from the oven, pour the remaining juice into the gravy bowl, and whisk to combine. Cut the meatloaf into 6 slices and serve with the gravy.

MAKE IT PALEO/DAIRY-FREE: Use dairy-free cheese or leave the cheese out and add extra vegetables. Omit the cream or substitute a nondairy milk alternative.

PER SERVING (1 slice)

Calories: 341; Total Fat: 25g; Protein: 25g; Total Carbs: 4g; Fiber: 1.5g; Net Carbs: 2.5g

ITALIAN MARINATED BAKED CHICKEN CAPRESE

SERVES 4 | PREP TIME: 20 MINUTES | COOK TIME: 1 HOUR

EGG-FREE · NUT-FREE

The trick to this recipe is to give the tomatoes a quick jaunt in the oven to caramelize a bit before you stuff them into the chicken. This cooks off the tomatoes' extra moisture, leaving flavor-packed morsels.

Coconut oil, for greasing

4 plum tomatoes

3 tablespoons extra-virgin olive oil, divided

Garlic salt

Freshly ground black pepper

10 fresh basil leaves, divided

4 (4-ounce) boneless, skinless chicken breasts

16 small herb-marinated mozzarella balls (about 4 ounces)

6 garlic cloves, minced

1 tablespoon Mediterranean Spice Blend (page 237)

1 tablespoon Italian seasoning

1. Preheat the oven to 450°F. Line a baking sheet with aluminum foil and grease it with oil.

2. Slice the plum tomatoes into ¼-inch-thick slices and place them flat on the prepared baking sheet in a single layer, not overlapping. Drizzle 1 tablespoon of olive oil over the top, then sprinkle with garlic salt and pepper. Chop about 5 basil leaves and sprinkle those over the top of the tomatoes as well. Bake for 20 minutes, then remove from the oven and let cool.

3. Pound the chicken breasts to about a 1-inch thickness, and then cut a horizontal slit into each to form a pocket.

4. Place the remaining fresh basil leaves inside the butterflied breasts, then top each breast with 4 mozzarella balls. Sprinkle equal amounts of garlic over each.

5. Use a fork to lift the tomatoes and lay them on top of the mozzarella. Drizzle the remaining 2 tablespoons of oil over the breasts, then sprinkle the Mediterranean spice blend, a decent dose of garlic salt, ground pepper, and Italian seasoning over the breasts.

6. Place the stuffed chicken breasts in a glass baking dish, or on a baking sheet lined with parchment paper. Bake uncovered for 40 minutes or until the internal temperature reaches 180°F. Serve right away with your favorite keto-friendly vegetables.

VARIATION TIP: If you don't have time to roast the tomatoes, you can use roasted red peppers (from a jar or pre-made) inside the chicken instead. You can also use chicken thighs instead of breasts.

PER SERVING (1 breast)

Calories: 380; Total Fat: 26g; Protein: 30g; Total Carbs: 6.5g; Fiber: 2g; Net Carbs: 4.5g

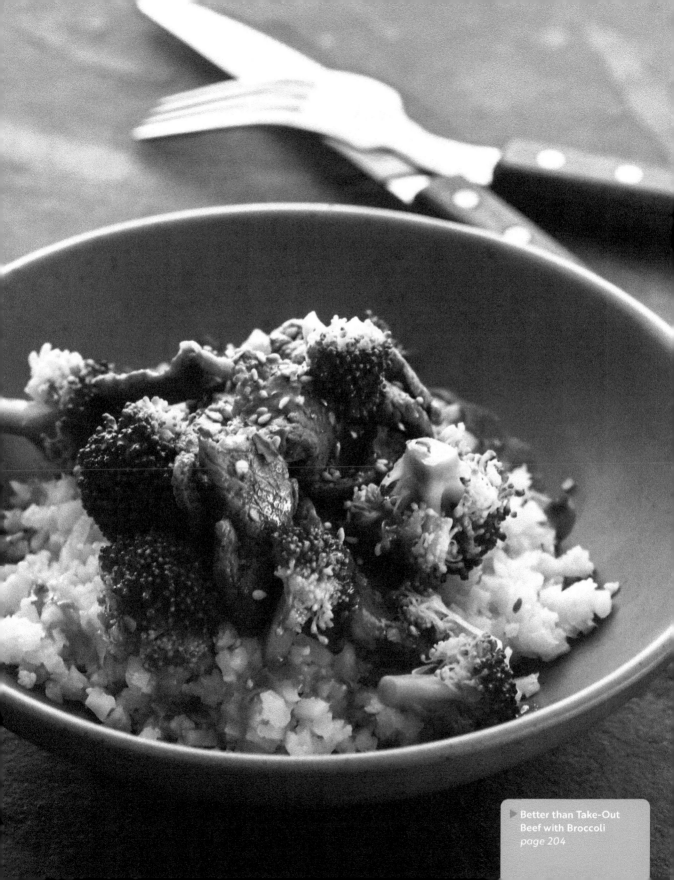

▶ Better than Take-Out
Beef with Broccoli
page 204

Pork, Beef, and Lamb

CRACK SLAW

SERVES 4 | PREP TIME: 5 MINUTES | COOK TIME: 35 MINUTES

EGG-FREE · NUT-FREE

I'm not sure where the name for this recipe came from but it's been circulating in the keto community for a while now. This is my version of "crack slaw" and it's a perfect one-pot meal that's a great option for lunch or dinner prep during the week.

2 tablespoons butter, ghee, or coconut oil

1 pound ground pork or sausage

1 small head green cabbage, shredded

2 tablespoons liquid or coconut aminos

1 tablespoon fish sauce

1 tablespoon coconut vinegar or apple cider vinegar

1 teaspoon garlic powder

1 teaspoon onion powder

¼ teaspoon ground ginger

Pinch red pepper flakes

Pinch sea salt

Pinch freshly ground black pepper

1 scallion, chopped

1. In a large skillet over medium heat, melt the butter or heat the oil and add the ground pork or sausage. Cook, stirring, until browned, 5 to 7 minutes. Add the shredded cabbage and mix to combine. Add the aminos, fish sauce, vinegar, garlic powder, onion powder, ginger, and red pepper flakes and mix well.

2. Simmer on low for 20 to 30 minutes, stirring occasionally, until the cabbage is cooked down and tender.

3. Season with salt and pepper and top with the chopped scallion.

4. Serve immediately or store in refrigerator for up to 1 week.

VARIATION TIP: You can substitute any ground meat of your choice or leave it out altogether and serve this as a yummy vegetable side dish.

PER SERVING

Calories: 356; Total Fat: 24g; Protein: 24g; Total Carbs: 11g; Fiber: 4g; Net Carbs: 7g

PORK RIND NACHOS

SERVES 1 | PREP TIME: 3 MINUTES | COOK TIME: 1 MINUTE

EGG-FREE · NUT-FREE · UNDER 30 MINUTES

Who doesn't love nachos? This is one of my go-to dinner or snack recipes when I don't feel like cooking or am just craving some crunch. It's ready in less than 5 minutes and satisfies any desire for a junk food binge. I like to use the Bacon's Heir or EPIC brand pork rinds and mix up the different flavor choices (barbecue is my fave). Feel free to swap out the pulled pork for any other type of cooked meat, or leave the meat out altogether and add some extra cheese.

2 ounces (about ¼ cup) Slow Cooker Pulled Pork (page 194)

2 cups (about 1 ounce) pork rinds

⅛ cup shredded Cheddar cheese

1 tablespoon salsa

1 tablespoon sour cream

5 pickled jalapeños slices (optional)

Pinch chili powder

1. Heat the pulled pork in the microwave for 30 to 60 seconds until heated through.

2. Place the pork rinds in an even layer on a microwave-safe plate. Layer the pulled pork on top and then sprinkle the Cheddar over the pork. Heat in the microwave for 20 to 30 seconds until the cheese is melted.

3. Remove from the microwave and top with salsa, sour cream, jalapeños (if using), and chili powder.

RECIPE TIP: Cooking for a crowd? Quadruple the recipe and bake in the oven on 350°F for 5 to 7 minutes or until the cheese is melted.

PER SERVING

Calories: 396; Total Fat: 28g; Protein: 34g; Total Carbs: 2g; Fiber: 0g; Net Carbs: 2g

SLOW COOKER PULLED PORK

MAKES 10 TO 12 CUPS SHREDDED PORK | PREP TIME: 5 MINUTES | COOK TIME: 8 TO 10 HOURS

EGG-FREE · NUT-FREE · PALEO/DAIRY-FREE · BULK PREP

This recipe is delicious on its own, but it's even better when it's paired with one of the sauces. Cooking for just one or two people? No problem. Freeze the leftovers and prepare the desired sauce when you're ready to serve.

FOR THE PULLED PORK

1 large onion, sliced

6 garlic cloves, smashed

1 tablespoon ground cumin

1 tablespoon chili powder

2 teaspoons sea salt

1 teaspoon freshly ground
  black pepper

½ teaspoon cayenne pepper (optional)

1 (4- to 6-pound) boneless pork
  shoulder (or 6 to 8 pounds bone-in)

2 cups Bone Broth (page 240)

PER SERVING (3 ounces, about ⅓ cup)

Calories: 224; Total Fat: 16g; Protein: 20g; Total Carbs: 0g;
Fiber: 0g; Net Carbs: 0g

TO MAKE THE PULLED PORK

1. Arrange the onion slices on the bottom of the slow cooker and scatter the garlic cloves over the top.

2. In a small bowl, whisk together the cumin, chili powder, salt, pepper, and cayenne (if using). Rub the spice mixture all over the pork shoulder and then place the meat on top of the onion and garlic in the slow cooker.

3. Pour the bone broth over the pork, cover, and cook on high for 2 hours. Reduce the heat to low and cook for another 6 hours until the meat is tender and falls apart easily. Do not lift the lid during cooking. Alternatively, you can cook on low for 8 to 10 hours.

4. Transfer the pork to a bowl, reserving the broth for the sauces, and shred it using two forks.

RECIPE TIP: If you don't have a slow cooker, you can use a large Dutch oven or roasting pan and cook the pork for 4 to 6 hours at 300°F until fork-tender.

Asian Fusion Sauce

1 cup reserved broth from cooking the pork, or beef broth

2 tablespoons liquid aminos or tamari

2 teaspoons coconut aminos

2 teaspoons coconut vinegar or apple cider vinegar

1 teaspoon chili paste

½ teaspoon garlic powder

¼ teaspoon ground ginger

Dash monk fruit or sweetener of choice

¼ teaspoon xanthan or guar gum, for thickening (optional)

PER SERVING (1 tablespoon)

Calories: 24; Total Fat: 1.5g; Protein: 1g; Total Carbs: 1.5g; Fiber: 0g; Net Carbs: 1.5g

Barbecue Sauce

1 cup reserved broth from cooking the pork, or beef broth

1 tablespoon tomato paste

1 tablespoon hot sauce

1 tablespoon yellow mustard

2 teaspoons coconut aminos

1 teaspoon garlic powder

1 teaspoon chili powder

Pinch sea salt

Pinch freshly ground black pepper

Dash monk fruit or sweetener of choice (optional)

¼ teaspoon xanthan or guar gum, for thickening (optional)

TO MAKE THE SAUCES

1. In a medium saucepan, whisk together all of the ingredients except for the xanthan gum, and simmer, whisking occasionally, over low to medium heat for 10 minutes or until thickened.

2. If desired, thicken the sauce by whisking in the xanthan gum.

RECIPE TIP: Depending on how flavorful your broth is, you may need to add additional salt and pepper to the sauces.

PER SERVING (1 tablespoon)

Calories: 28; Total Fat: 1.5g; Protein: 1.5g; Total Carbs: 2g; Fiber: 0.5g; Net Carbs: 1.5g

BACON MAC 'N' CHEESE

SERVES 6 | PREP TIME: 10 MINUTES | COOK TIME: 20 MINUTES

EGG-FREE · NUT-FREE · UNDER 30 MINUTES

Comfort food at its finest, without the guilt! Creamy, cheesy, with a touch of crunch, this dish is everything you need to satisfy those comfort food cravings while still keeping your goals in check. This recipe definitely makes the cut for my top five favorites in this book.

1 cauliflower head, chopped into small pieces (about 4 cups)

6 bacon slices

½ cup heavy (whipping) cream

3 ounces cream cheese, cut into cubes

1½ cups shredded sharp Cheddar cheese

2 teaspoons Dijon or yellow mustard

1 teaspoon garlic powder

1 teaspoon onion powder

1 teaspoon paprika

¼ teaspoon cayenne pepper

Sea salt

Freshly ground black pepper

Chopped fresh parsley (optional)

1. In a large microwave-safe dish, cook the cauliflower florets on high for 15 to 20 minutes until tender. Alternatively, you can steam the cauliflower on the stovetop until tender. If using frozen cauliflower, follow the package instructions for steaming, but be careful not to overcook.

2. Meanwhile, in a large skillet, cook the bacon over medium-high heat for 5 to 7 minutes until crisp. Transfer to a paper towel and let cool. Reserve the bacon grease for the sauce, if desired.

3. While the bacon and cauliflower are cooking, prepare the cheese sauce. In a large saucepan over medium-low heat, bring the cream to a simmer. Add the cream cheese and cook, whisking, until the cream cheese melts.

4. Add the Cheddar, mustard, garlic powder, onion powder, paprika, and cayenne. Reduce the heat to low and cook, whisking, until the Cheddar melts. Continue to cook on low heat, whisking constantly, for 2 to 3 minutes more until the sauce thickens.

5. Remove the pan from the heat and season with salt and pepper. The sauce will be thick, but once you add the cauliflower, it will thin out a bit.

6. Drain any excess liquid from the cauliflower and stir it into the cheese sauce. Crumble in the bacon and stir to combine. Serve immediately, garnished with parsley (if using).

INGREDIENT TIP: Add 1 or 2 tablespoons of the leftover bacon grease to the cheese sauce to give it another flavor boost.

RECIPE TIP: If you like baked mac 'n' cheese with a crunchy topping, just add the cauliflower mixture to a greased baking dish, sprinkle with crushed pork rinds and Parmesan cheese, and bake at 350°F for 10 to 15 minutes until the cheese melts and the topping browns.

PER SERVING (about 1 cup)

Calories: 307; Total Fat: 25g; Protein: 13g; Total Carbs: 7.5g; Fiber: 2.5g; Net Carbs: 5g

PORK TENDERLOIN WITH CREAMY HORSERADISH SAUCE

SERVES 4 | PREP TIME: 5 MINUTES | COOK TIME: 25 MINUTES

EGG-FREE · NUT-FREE · PALEO/DAIRY-FREE OPTION · UNDER 30 MINUTES

Pork tenderloin is one of those dishes that can either be super juicy and flavorful or bland and dried out. This recipe keeps things simple while still achieving a tender roast paired with a slightly spicy, decadent sauce. The horseradish and cayenne make this sauce very flavorful, but you can adjust the amounts depending on your preference.

FOR THE PORK

1 pork tenderloin (about 1 pound)

1 teaspoon garlic powder

1 teaspoon onion powder

1 teaspoon sea salt

½ teaspoon freshly ground black pepper

1 tablespoon avocado or coconut oil or lard

½ cup Bone Broth (page 240)

2 tablespoons butter or ghee

2 tablespoons heavy (whipping) cream

1 tablespoon Dijon mustard

1 tablespoon spicy horseradish

¼ teaspoon cayenne pepper

1 teaspoon gelatin or ⅛ teaspoon xanthan or guar gum, to thicken (optional)

1. Season the pork with the garlic powder, onion powder, salt, and pepper.

2. In a large skillet, heat the oil or lard over medium-high heat. Add the pork and brown for 3 to 4 minutes on one side. Rotate the pork one-third of the way and brown for another 3 to 4 minutes. Repeat for the last side (total of 9 to 12 minutes browning time).

3. Remove the pork to a plate to rest. It will not be cooked all the way through yet, which is okay because it will cook more in the sauce.

4. Place the skillet back on the stove over medium-high heat. Add the bone broth and bring to a boil, scraping the drippings and brown bits off the bottom of the skillet.

5. Reduce the heat to medium and whisk in the butter, cream, mustard, horseradish, cayenne, and gelatin (if using). Let simmer, whisking often, for 5 minutes.

6. Once the sauce begins to thicken, cut the pork into ½-inch-thick pieces and return them to the skillet. Coat the meat with the sauce and let simmer for another 5 minutes until the pork is cooked through.

MAKE IT PALEO/DAIRY-FREE: Replace the heavy cream with full-fat coconut milk or nondairy milk of choice. Use ghee if tolerated or replace with beef tallow or lard.

PER SERVING

Calories: 243; Total Fat: 15g; Protein: 25g; Total Carbs: 2g; Fiber: 0.5g; Net Carbs: 1.5g

CHESOS (CHEESE SHELL TACOS) CARNITAS

SERVES 4 | PREP TIME: 10 MINUTES | COOK TIME: 10 MINUTES

EGG-FREE · NUT-FREE · UNDER 30 MINUTES

Who needs corn or flour when you can make a shell out of pure cheese? These cheese shell tacos are a complete game changer and very simple to make. Whether you're stuffing them with carnitas, chorizo, ground beef, or shrimp, they are sure to be a crowd-pleaser.

2 cups shredded Cheddar cheese

2 cups (about 8 ounces) Slow Cooker Pulled Pork (page 194)

2 tablespoons Mexican Spice Blend (page 237)

TOPPING SUGGESTIONS

Avocado slices

Sour cream

Salsa

Jalapeños

Chopped onion

Fresh cilantro

Hot sauce

1. Preheat the oven to 400°F. Line one large (or two medium) baking sheets with parchment paper or a silicone mat.

2. Place ¼-cup piles of shredded cheese on the prepared baking sheet, forming them into even circles. Leave several inches between the piles to ensure the cheese shells don't melt together.

3. Bake for 6 to 8 minutes until the cheese melts and the edges are lightly browned.

4. While the cheese is baking, wrap the handle of two or three wooden spoons or skewers with aluminum foil and balance each one between two cans or cups.

5. Remove the cheese from the oven and let cool for 3 minutes. Using a spatula, drape each cheese round over one of the foil handles or skewers. The cheese will harden into a shell shape as it sets, about 10 minutes.

6. While the chesos are hardening, toss the pork in the Mexican spice blend and warm it in the microwave or oven.

7. Fill each cheese shell with ¼ cup of pork and add your desired toppings.

RECIPE TIP: You can also make individual chesos in the microwave by placing the cheese on a piece of parchment paper and microwaving for 1 minute, then follow the same steps after cooling as listed above.

PER SERVING (2 taco shells with ¼ cup carnitas, not including toppings)

Calories: 385; Total Fat: 29g; Protein: 28g; Total Carbs: 3g; Fiber: 1g; Net Carbs: 2g

PORK FRIED CAULIFLOWER RICE

SERVES 4 | PREP TIME: 10 MINUTES | COOK TIME: 20 MINUTES

EGG-FREE · NUT-FREE · PALEO/DAIRY-FREE · UNDER 30 MINUTES

Don't try to trick yourself into thinking your Chinese take-out is healthy because it's mostly meat and veggies. Instead, throw together this quick and easy skillet meal that will curb all your cravings.

1 pound ground pork

Sea salt

Freshly ground black pepper

3 tablespoons toasted sesame oil

3 cups thinly sliced cabbage

1 cup chopped broccoli

1 red bell pepper, cored and chopped

1 garlic clove, minced

1½ cups riced cauliflower

1 tablespoon sriracha

2 tablespoons liquid aminos or tamari

1 teaspoon rice wine vinegar

1 teaspoon sesame seeds, for garnish

1. Heat a medium skillet over medium-high heat. Add the pork and sprinkle generously with salt and pepper. Cook, stirring frequently, until browned, about 10 minutes. Remove the meat from the skillet.

2. Reduce the heat to medium and add the sesame oil to the skillet along with the cabbage, broccoli, bell pepper, riced cauliflower, and garlic. Cook for about 5 minutes until slightly softened, then add the sriracha, liquid aminos, and vinegar and mix well.

3. Return the browned pork to the skillet. Simmer together for about 5 minutes more until the cabbage is crisp-tender. Season with salt and pepper, then garnish with the sesame seeds and serve right away.

VARIATION TIP: To make prep quicker, buy the pre-riced cauliflower and bagged coleslaw mix at your grocery store. Either fresh or frozen is fine because the moisture in the frozen cauliflower will cook off in the skillet. The same goes for the cabbage. You can make this quickly with a bagged coleslaw or broccoli slaw mix.

PER SERVING

Calories: 460; Total Fat: 36g; Protein: 23g; Total Carbs: 11g; Fiber: 5g; Net Carbs: 6g

LEMON BUTTER PORK CHOPS

SERVES 4 | PREP TIME: 5 MINUTES | COOK TIME: 25 MINUTES

EGG-FREE · NUT-FREE · UNDER 30 MINUTES

This simple and delicious lemon butter dish is great for a quick meal that tastes like something you could order at a restaurant. It's excellent served alone, or atop hot, salted, and peppered zoodles. Green beans and spinach are great side dishes for this recipe because they pair beautifully with the sauce.

½ teaspoon sea salt

1 teaspoon lemon-pepper seasoning

1 teaspoon garlic powder

½ teaspoon dried thyme

4 (4-ounce) boneless pork chops

5 tablespoons butter, divided

¼ cup Bone Broth (page 240)

2 tablespoons freshly squeezed
   lemon juice

1 tablespoon minced garlic

½ cup heavy (whipping) cream

1. In a small bowl, stir together the salt, lemon-pepper seasoning, garlic powder, and thyme. Rub the spice mixture all over the pork chops.

2. Heat a skillet over medium-high heat and melt 2 tablespoons of butter. Add the pork chops and cook for at least 5 minutes on each side until they are cooked through. Remove the chops from the pan.

3. Reduce the heat to medium-low. Add the bone broth, lemon juice, garlic, and the remaining 3 tablespoons of butter. Add the pork chops and simmer for about 15 minutes, adding the cream 1 tablespoon at a time every few minutes, until the sauce thickens.

4. Remove from the heat and serve.

VARIATION TIP: This recipe works great with all kinds of protein, so feel free to substitute some pounded chicken breasts or even shrimp for the pork chops.

PER SERVING

Calories: 379; Total Fat: 29g; Protein: 27g; Total Carbs: 2.5g; Fiber: 0g; Net Carbs: 2.5g

CREAMY PORK MARSALA

SERVES 4 | PREP TIME: 5 MINUTES | COOK TIME: 30 MINUTES

EGG-FREE · NUT-FREE · PALEO/DAIRY-FREE OPTION

If you've never made Marsala sauce before, it might sound intimidating, but you can create a simple sauce with just a few ingredients and one skillet. Marsala wine is a fortified wine from Sicily. It's a bit sweet, like a sherry. If you don't have Marsala, you can use sherry or any white wine that is a bit on the sweet side.

4 (4-ounce) boneless pork cutlets

Salt

Freshly ground black pepper

4 tablespoons butter, divided

8 ounces sliced mushrooms (cremini, portabella, button, or other)

4 ounces prosciutto, chopped

1 garlic clove, minced

½ cup Marsala cooking wine

½ cup Bone Broth (page 240)

1 teaspoon chopped fresh thyme

½ teaspoon xanthan or guar gum, to thicken (optional)

Chopped fresh parsley, for garnish

1. Sprinkle the cutlets with salt and pepper.

2. Heat a large skillet over medium-high heat and melt 2 tablespoons of butter. Add the cutlets and cook for at least 5 minutes on each side until cooked through. Remove the cutlets from the skillet.

3. Reduce the heat to medium-low and add the remaining 2 tablespoons of butter. Add the mushrooms, prosciutto, and garlic, and cook, stirring frequently, until the mushrooms brown, about 5 minutes.

4. Add the wine, bone broth, and thyme. Simmer for about 15 minutes until the sauce thickens. Add the xanthan gum (if using), to thicken the sauce even more. Return the pork to the skillet and raise the heat to medium-high. Cook until the cutlets are heated through.

5. Serve garnished with parsley.

MAKE IT PALEO/DAIRY-FREE: Replace the butter with ghee or coconut oil.

VARIATION TIP: This sauce is excellent with crispy chicken thighs as well. Simply cook them in the oven, then broil them until the skin is crispy and serve atop the sauce.

PER SERVING

Calories: 339; Total Fat: 19g; Protein: 36g; Total Carbs: 6g; Fiber: 0.5g; Net Carbs: 5.5g

BETTER THAN TAKE-OUT BEEF WITH BROCCOLI

SERVES 4 | PREP TIME: 10 MINUTES, PLUS AT LEAST 4 HOURS TO MARINATE |
COOK TIME: 20 MINUTES

EGG-FREE · NUT-FREE · PALEO/DAIRY-FREE

Chinese food was probably one of my favorite foods growing up. I've always been a sucker for beef and broccoli, so I had to make a keto version. This beef and broccoli dish is paired with a thick, flavorful sauce that will kick your craving for Chinese take-out. Serve it over cauliflower rice or shirataki noodles to absorb all that tasty marinade.

FOR THE MARINADE

3 tablespoons coconut aminos (or
    2 tablespoons liquid aminos)

2 tablespoons coconut oil, melted

2 tablespoons toasted sesame oil

2 tablespoons fish sauce

1 tablespoon coconut vinegar
    or apple cider vinegar

1 teaspoon onion powder

1 teaspoon garlic powder

½ teaspoon ground ginger

¼ teaspoon red pepper flakes

FOR THE BEEF AND BROCCOLI

1 pound beef sirloin or flank, sliced
    thinly across the grain

2 cups broccoli florets

1 tablespoon coconut oil

2 garlic cloves, minced

½ teaspoon sea salt

¼ teaspoon freshly ground
    black pepper

1 tablespoon toasted sesame seeds
    (optional)

TO MAKE THE MARINADE

In a medium bowl, whisk together the coconut aminos, coconut oil, sesame oil, fish sauce, vinegar, onion powder, garlic powder, ginger, and red pepper flakes.

TO MAKE THE BEEF AND BROCCOLI

1. In a large plastic bag or medium bowl, pour one-third of the marinade over the beef and let marinate in the refrigerator for a few hours or overnight. Save the rest of the marinade in a small container to use for the sauce.

2. In a large pot, steam the broccoli until just tender. Transfer to a bowl with ice and cold water to stop the cooking. Drain and set aside.

3. In a large skillet or wok, heat the coconut oil over high heat. Remove the beef from the marinade (discard the marinade) and add the beef to the skillet. Let brown for 2 to 3 minutes. Flip the meat and cook for another 2 to 3 minutes.

4. Add the garlic, salt, and pepper and stir to combine.

5. Add the cooked broccoli florets and the reserved marinade. Stir well and let simmer on medium-low heat for 5 to 10 minutes or until the sauce thickens and the meat is cooked through. Top with sesame seeds (if using).

VARIATION TIP: Feel free to swap the sirloin for ribeye, ground beef, or other meat of choice.

RECIPE TIP: For a thicker sauce, stir in ½ to 1 teaspoon xanthan or guar gum at the end of cooking.

PER SERVING

Calories: 356; Total Fat: 24g; Protein: 29g; Total Carbs: 6g; Fiber: 1.5g; Net Carbs: 4.5g

SPECIAL CHORIZO WITH AVOCADO CREMA

SERVES 4 | PREP TIME: 5 MINUTES | COOK TIME: 10 MINUTES

EGG-FREE · NUT-FREE · PALEO/DAIRY-FREE OPTION · UNDER 30 MINUTES

Chorizo is a Mexican sausage made with a unique blend of spices. It is flavorful on its own, but we'll kick it up a notch with two secret ingredients: nutmeg and cinnamon. The sweetness of these spices paired with the spicy chorizo will delight your taste buds. Add the creamy, tangy avocado crema and you'll be in heaven. Serve the chorizo in butter lettuce cups or over cauliflower rice topped with shredded cheese, salsa, green onions, and hot sauce.

1 pound loose chorizo

¼ teaspoon ground nutmeg

½ teaspoon ground cinnamon

1¼ teaspoons sea salt, divided

¾ teaspoon freshly ground black pepper, divided

1 avocado, mashed

¼ cup sour cream

Juice of ½ lime

1 teaspoon chili powder

1. In a medium skillet over medium heat, combine the chorizo, nutmeg, cinnamon, 1 teaspoon of salt, and ¼ teaspoon of pepper and cook, stirring frequently, until browned and cooked through, 5 to 7 minutes.

2. Meanwhile, in a small bowl, stir together the avocado, sour cream, lime juice, chili powder, the remaining ¼ teaspoon of salt, and the remaining ¼ teaspoon of pepper.

3. Serve the chorizo with the crema drizzled over it.

MAKE IT PALEO/DAIRY-FREE: Replace the sour cream in the crema with 2 tablespoons of unsweetened coconut milk or cream.

INGREDIENT TIP: Check the nutritional label on your chorizo to make sure it has minimal carbs and no added sugars or other questionable ingredients.

PER SERVING (3 ounces cooked chorizo)

Calories: 256; Total Fat: 20g; Protein: 18g; Total Carbs: 1g; Fiber: 0g; Net Carbs: 1g

PER SERVING (about 2 tablespoons Avocado Crema)

Calories: 94; Total Fat: 8g; Protein: 1g; Total Carbs: 4.5g; Fiber: 3g; Net Carbs: 1.5g

MEATZA PIZZA

SERVES 4 | PREP TIME: 5 MINUTES | COOK TIME: 25 MINUTES

NUT-FREE · PALEO/DAIRY-FREE · UNDER 30 MINUTES

This is one of those busy weeknight recipes that takes absolutely no brainpower to throw together. If you have any type of ground meat in the refrigerator, all you have to do is add some spices, form it into a pizza, and add your favorite toppings. It's quick, easy, and satisfies that pizza craving with very few carbs.

1 pound ground beef

1 large egg

1 tablespoon Italian seasoning

1 teaspoon onion powder

1 teaspoon garlic powder

1 teaspoon sea salt

½ teaspoon freshly ground black pepper

TOPPING SUGGESTIONS

¼ cup low-sugar pizza sauce

2 tablespoons Easy Peasy Garlicky Pesto (page 245)

Pepperoni or prosciutto slices

1 cup sautéed vegetables

½ cup shredded cheese

1. Preheat the oven to 400°F.
2. In a large bowl, mix together the ground beef, egg, Italian seasoning, onion powder, and garlic powder.
3. In a cast iron skillet or other oven-safe skillet, form the meat mixture into a round pizza crust shape, about ½- to 1-inch thick.
4. Bake for 15 to 20 minutes until the meat is browned and cooked through.
5. Remove the meat from the oven and drain off any excess liquid from the skillet. Add the toppings to the meat and return to the oven for 3 to 5 minutes to heat the toppings.
6. Let cool for 5 minutes and serve.

VARIATION TIP: Substitute ground pork, turkey, chicken, lamb, sausage, or a combination of a few different meats for the ground beef. Feel free to mix up the spices for different flavor combinations.

PER SERVING (¼ Meatza without toppings)

Calories: 308; Total Fat: 24g; Protein: 21g; Total Carbs: 2g; Fiber: 1g; Net Carbs: 1g

BREAKFAST BURGER IN A LETTUCE BUN

SERVES 4 | PREP TIME: 10 MINUTES | COOK TIME: 15 MINUTES

NUT-FREE · UNDER 30 MINUTES

Once you ditch the burger bun for some crunchy lettuce, you'll forget why you ever needed it. A lettuce bun brings a freshness to this dish and ditches that heavy belly you get from a big roll. This burger comes with a satisfying serving of bacon and egg on top to complete the meal for breakfast or any time of day.

1 pound ground beef, formed into 4 burger patties

½ teaspoon onion powder

½ teaspoon garlic powder

½ teaspoon salt

¼ teaspoon freshly ground black pepper

4 bacon slices

8 large lettuce leaves

4 Cheddar cheese slices

4 eggs

1. Sprinkle the beef patties generously with the onion powder, garlic powder, salt, and pepper. Use your thumb to press a dimple into the middle of each patty, which will help them keep a flat shape as they cook.

2. Heat a large skillet over medium-high heat and cook the bacon for 5 to 7 minutes until crisp. Transfer to a paper towel, leaving the bacon grease in the skillet.

3. Cook the burger patties in the bacon grease in the skillet, covered, over medium-high heat for 2 to 4 minutes

on each side, depending on how you like your burgers cooked.

4. Add a slice of cheese to each patty, cover the skillet, and let cook for another 30 seconds or so until the cheese is melted. Remove the burgers from the skillet.

5. Add the eggs to the skillet and cook over medium-high heat for just about 30 seconds for a soft sunny-side-up doneness. Don't flip them!

6. On a plate, place 1 large lettuce leaf, topped by a burger patty, 1 slice of bacon, and 1 egg. Season with salt and pepper.

7. Top with 1 more lettuce leaf and serve immediately.

VARIATION TIP: The size of the burger is really up to you. You can make smaller patties and enjoy them as sliders, which are better stacked with a slice of cheese in between them.

PER SERVING

Calories: 492; Total Fat: 38g; Protein: 34g; Total Carbs: 3.5g; Fiber: 1.5g; Net Carbs: 2g

SKIRT STEAK WITH FRESH GARDEN HERB BUTTER

SERVES 4 | PREP TIME: 20 MINUTES | COOK TIME: 10 MINUTES

EGG-FREE · NUT-FREE · UNDER 30 MINUTES

Fresh herbs are important for this recipe, as the dried stuff just won't deliver the same punch. If you don't have an herb garden, no problem, get your fresh herbs from the produce section of your grocery store. This recipe makes a big batch of fresh herb butter for you to save and devour on many steaks to come.

FOR THE BUTTER

1½ cups (3 sticks) butter,
    at room temperature

1 tablespoon minced garlic

½ cup finely chopped basil

1 tablespoon chopped parsley

1 tablespoon minced chives

1½ teaspoons sea salt

FOR THE STEAK

1 pound skirt steak, cut into
    4 separate steaks

1 teaspoon garlic powder

1 teaspoon sea salt

½ teaspoon freshly ground pepper

1 tablespoon coconut oil or other
    cooking fat

VARIATION TIP: You can cook the steak however you want. In fact, they're great done on the grill.

PER SERVING (1 steak plus 1 tablespoon herb butter)

Calories: 376; Total Fat: 32g; Protein: 21g; Total Carbs: 1g; Fiber: 0g; Net Carbs: 1g

TO MAKE THE BUTTER

In a medium bowl, combine the butter with the garlic, basil, parsley, chives, and salt and stir until the mixture is well combined and smooth. Set aside ¼ cup of the mixture to use for the steak, and refrigerate the rest in an airtight container, or rolled into a log wrapped in parchment paper. Store the butter in the refrigerator for up to 1 week or in the freezer for up to 3 months.

TO MAKE THE STEAK

1. Season the steak generously with the garlic powder, salt, and pepper, then let sit at room temperature for 10 to 15 minutes.

2. Oil a cast iron skillet and heat it over medium-high heat.

3. Cook each steak in the pan for 2 to 6 minutes on each side, depending on how you like your steak.

4. Serve hot, each steak topped with 1 tablespoon of the butter. Let the butter melt, then enjoy!

BEEF STROGANOFF

SERVES 6 | PREP TIME: 10 MINUTES | COOK TIME: 35 MINUTES

EGG-FREE · NUT-FREE · PALEO/DAIRY-FREE OPTION · BULK PREP

I love making a big batch of this beef stroganoff recipe for the week. It's creamy, satisfying, and goes great over sautéed cabbage, zoodles, or cauliflower rice for an easy meal. You could even swap the sirloin for ground beef to make it more budget-friendly.

1 tablespoon coconut oil, lard, or other cooking fat

1½ pounds beef sirloin, cut against the grain into thin strips

½ teaspoon sea salt, plus additional

¼ teaspoon freshly ground black pepper, plus additional

2 tablespoons butter or ghee

½ cup chopped onion

3 garlic cloves, minced

3 cups sliced mushrooms (about 8 ounces)

1 teaspoon dried oregano

⅛ teaspoon cayenne pepper (optional)

1 cup Bone Broth (page 240)

½ cup heavy (whipping) cream

½ cup sour cream

½ to 1 teaspoon xanthan or guar gum, for thickening

½ teaspoon garlic powder

½ teaspoon onion powder

Chopped fresh parsley, for garnish (optional)

1. In a large skillet, heat the oil over medium-high heat.

2. Season the beef strips with the salt and pepper and then add half of the beef to the pot and cook for 1 to 2 minutes on each side, just until browned. Remove to a large bowl and repeat with the remaining beef.

3. Once all the beef is browned and removed to the bowl, reduce the heat to medium and add the butter to the skillet along with the onion, garlic, and mushrooms. Season with the oregano and cayenne (if using). Season with a bit more salt and pepper. Cook the onions and mushrooms for 7 to 10 minutes, stirring occasionally, until tender. Remove the onion, mushrooms, and garlic to the bowl with the beef.

4. Add the bone broth to the skillet and bring to a boil. Once boiling, reduce the heat to low and slowly whisk in the cream, sour cream, xanthan or guar gum, garlic powder, and onion powder. Stir for 3 to 5 minutes until the broth starts to thicken.

5. Return the beef and vegetable mixture to the pot. Cook on low for another 5 to 10 minutes until the beef is cooked through and the sauce is thickened. Garnish with parsley (if using) and serve.

MAKE IT PALEO/DAIRY-FREE: Replace the heavy cream with ⅓ cup full-fat coconut milk and leave out the sour cream.

PER SERVING

Calories: 326; Total Fat: 22g; Protein: 27g; Total Carbs: 5g; Fiber: 1g; Net Carbs: 4g

SHEPHERD'S PIE WITH CAULIFLOWER MASH

SERVES 8 | PREP TIME: 20 MINUTES | COOK TIME: 30 MINUTES

EGG-FREE · NUT-FREE · PALEO/DAIRY-FREE OPTION · BULK PREP

I made this dish for my roommate a while ago and she had no idea that I switched out the traditional mashed potatoes for cauliflower mash. The texture is so similar, and as long as you season the cauliflower mash well, I promise you won't even miss the potatoes. Feel free to swap the mushrooms for other low-carb veggies like spinach, asparagus, or celery.

6 cups fresh or frozen cauliflower florets or rice

2 pounds ground beef or lamb

1 tablespoon butter or ghee, plus ¼ cup, melted

½ cup chopped onion

3 garlic cloves, minced

2 tablespoons Italian seasoning

1 tablespoon tomato paste

2 cups chopped mushrooms

2 teaspoons sea salt, divided

1 teaspoon freshly ground black pepper, divided

4 ounces cream cheese, at room temperature

1 tablespoon Italian seasoning

1 teaspoon garlic powder

½ cup grated Parmesan or white Cheddar cheese

1. Preheat the oven to 375°F.

2. Place the cauliflower in a microwave-safe dish and cook on high for 6 to 8 minutes if using frozen (10 to 15 minutes if using fresh), until tender. Transfer to a colander to drain.

3. Meanwhile, in a large skillet over medium heat, cook the ground meat until browned, 5 to 7 minutes. Drain the excess liquid and transfer the meat to a bowl.

4. In the same skillet, melt 1 tablespoon of butter and add the onion. Cook for 3 minutes over medium-high heat. Add the garlic, Italian seasoning, tomato paste, mushrooms, 1 teaspoon of salt, and ½ teaspoon of pepper and cook for another 5 to 8 minutes until the mushrooms are cooked down.

5. While the mushrooms are cooking, strain off any excess liquid from the cauliflower and add it to a blender or food processor with the remaining ¼ cup of melted butter, cream cheese, Italian seasoning, garlic powder, remaining 1 teaspoon of salt, and remaining ½ teaspoon of pepper. Blend until smooth. Taste and adjust the seasoning.

6. Return the meat to the skillet with the mushrooms and onions and stir well. Transfer the meat mixture to a 9-by-13-inch baking dish. Spoon the cauliflower mixture over the top and smooth it into an even layer. Sprinkle with the cheese and bake for 20 minutes.

7. Let cool and cut into 8 squares.

MAKE IT PALEO/DAIRY-FREE: For the topping, replace the cream cheese with full-fat coconut milk and sprinkle with nutritional yeast instead of cheese.

PER SERVING

Calories: 395; Total Fat: 27g; Protein: 30g; Total Carbs: 8g; Fiber: 3g; Net Carbs: 5g

SLOW COOKER LAMB CURRY

MAKES 10 TO 12 CUPS SHREDDED LAMB | PREP TIME: 5 MINUTES | COOK TIME: 8 TO 10 HOURS

EGG-FREE · NUT-FREE · BULK PREP

This is a throw it all in, set it, and forget it recipe. The flavor combination is spectacular and this recipe makes enough to store in the freezer for several meals throughout the coming months. Pair with cauliflower or shirataki rice for a flavorful and filling meal.

1 large onion, cut into thick slices

6 garlic cloves, smashed

2 tablespoons Indian Spice Blend (page 236), divided

2 teaspoons sea salt

1 teaspoon freshly ground black pepper

1 (4- to 6-pound) boneless leg of lamb or shoulder (or 6 to 8 pounds bone-in)

1 (14-ounce) can unsweetened coconut milk

3 tablespoons tomato paste

1 (2-inch) piece fresh ginger, peeled

2 tablespoons ghee or butter

⅛ teaspoon cayenne pepper (or more if you like spice)

½ to 1 teaspoon xanthan or guar gum

1. Arrange the onion slices on the bottom of the slow cooker and scatter the smashed garlic cloves on top.

2. Rub 1 tablespoon of the Indian spice blend, and the salt and pepper all over the lamb and place it on top of the onion and garlic.

3. In a medium bowl, whisk together the coconut milk and tomato paste. Add the mixture along with the ginger to the slow cooker.

4. Cover and cook on high for 2 hours and then turn the heat to low and cook for another 6 hours or until the meat is tender and falls apart easily. Do not lift the lid during cooking. You can also cook on low for 8 to 10 hours.

5. When the meat is tender and begins to fall apart, transfer it to a bowl and shred it using two forks.

6. Using a slotted spoon, remove the onions, garlic, and ginger from the slow cooker to a bowl and set aside. The amount of liquid left in the slow cooker will vary but it should come out to about 5 cups (more or less depending on the size of the leg of lamb).

7. In a large saucepan, melt the ghee over medium-high heat. Pour the liquid from the slow cooker into the pan with the ghee and bring to a boil. Once boiling, reduce the heat to medium-low and whisk in the remaining 1 tablespoon of the spice blend, the cayenne, and xanthan gum. Let simmer for 10 to 15 minutes, whisking occasionally, until the sauce is reduced and thickened. The liquid should reduce by about 1 cup, leaving you with about 4 cups of sauce. Serve the sauce over the lamb and garnish with the cooked onions.

8. To store, divide the lamb into airtight containers and store in the refrigerator for up to 1 week or in the freezer for up to 3 months. Divide the sauce into glass storage containers, filling them only three-quarters full, to allow room for the liquid to expand as it freezes, and store in the freezer for up to 3 months. Defrost the sauce to enjoy with the lamb or use it to jazz up another meat and vegetable dish.

RECIPE TIP: If you don't have a slow cooker, you can use a large Dutch oven or roasting pan and cook the lamb for 4 to 6 hours at 300°F or until fork-tender.

PER SERVING (about ⅓ cup cooked portion)

Calories: 214; Total Fat: 14g; Protein: 22g; Total Carbs: 0g; Fiber: 0g; Net Carbs: 0g

PER SERVING (about ¼ cup sauce)

Calories: 73; Total Fat: 7g; Protein: 1g; Total Carbs: 1.5g; Fiber: 0g; Net Carbs: 1.5g

LAMB DOGS WITH TZATZIKI

SERVES 10 | PREP TIME: 15 MINUTES | COOK TIME: 25 MINUTES

NUT-FREE · PALEO/DAIRY-FREE OPTION · BULK PREP

An adult twist on a kid's classic, these lamb dogs are packed with flavor and pair great with the tangy tzatziki. Instead of baking the lamb dogs, you can grill them or cook them in a skillet with a tablespoon of butter or oil, rotating to brown each side. Serve with Zesty Roasted Broccoli (page 227) or a simple Greek side salad for a complete meal.

FOR THE TZATZIKI

½ medium cucumber, peeled and grated on the large holes of a box grater

1 cup full-fat plain Greek yogurt

1 tablespoon extra-virgin olive oil

1 tablespoon chopped fresh dill (or ½ teaspoon dried dill weed)

1 teaspoon freshly squeezed lemon juice

1 garlic clove, minced (or ½ teaspoon garlic powder)

½ teaspoon sea salt

¼ teaspoon freshly ground black pepper

FOR THE LAMB DOGS

Oil or cooking spray, for greasing

2 pounds ground lamb (or a 50-50 mix of lamb and beef)

2 eggs

2 tablespoons Mediterranean Spice Blend (page 237) or Italian seasoning

2 tablespoons extra-virgin olive oil

2 scallions, finely chopped

¼ cup chopped fresh mint (optional)

2 teaspoons lemon-pepper seasoning

1 teaspoon garlic powder

1 teaspoon sea salt

½ teaspoon freshly ground black pepper

TO MAKE THE TZATZIKI

1. Wrap the grated cucumber in a clean dishtowel and squeeze out as much liquid as possible.

2. In a small bowl, whisk together the cucumber, yogurt, oil, dill, lemon juice, garlic, salt, and pepper.

3. Cover and chill in the refrigerator while you prepare the lamb dogs.

TO MAKE THE LAMB DOGS

1. Preheat the oven to 350°F. Line a baking sheet with aluminum foil and a baking rack. Grease or spray the rack with oil to prevent the lamb from sticking.

2. In a large bowl, mix together the ground meat, eggs, Mediterranean spice blend, oil, scallions, mint (if using), lemon-pepper seasoning, garlic powder, salt, and pepper.

3. Divide the meat mixture into 10 equal portions. The easiest way to do this is to form the mixture into one large, flat rectangle. Score it with your hand down the middle lengthwise and then score it 4 more times in the opposite direction so that you end up with 10 squares. Form each portion into a log (or hot dog shape) and place on the prepared baking rack.

4. Bake for 20 to 25 minutes until browned and cooked through.

5. Serve the lamb dogs topped with the sauce.

MAKE IT PALEO/DAIRY-FREE: Substitute coconut yogurt for the Greek yogurt (or use coconut kefir and add ⅛ teaspoon xanthan or guar gum to thicken).

PER SERVING (1 lamb dog)

Calories: 219; Total Fat: 15g; Protein: 20g; Total Carbs: 1g; Fiber: 0g; Net Carbs: 1g

PER SERVING (1 tablespoon tzatziki)

Calories: 30; Total Fat: 2g; Protein: 2g; Total Carbs: 1g; Fiber: 0g; Net Carbs: 1g

KETO BURRITO BOWL

SERVES 4 | PREP TIME: 10 MINUTES | COOK TIME: 30 MINUTES

EGG-FREE · NUT-FREE · PALEO/DAIRY-FREE OPTION

This burrito bowl is so simple to throw together and the cauliflower rice is the perfect substitute for traditional rice. Add a side of Keto Refried "Beans" (page 224) to jazz it up even more.

1 pound ground beef

1½ tablespoons Mexican Spice Blend (page 237), divided

2 teaspoons sea salt, divided

1 teaspoon freshly ground black pepper, divided

1 tablespoon butter or ghee

¼ cup chopped onion

2 garlic cloves, minced

4 cups fresh or frozen cauliflower rice

OPTIONAL TOPPINGS

Shredded cheese

Low-sugar salsa

Sour cream

Avocado slices

Hot sauce

Jalapeños

1. In a large skillet over medium heat, cook the beef with 1 tablespoon of Mexican spice blend, 1 teaspoon of salt, and ½ teaspoon of pepper, stirring frequently, until browned, 5 to 7 minutes.

2. In another large skillet over medium heat, melt the butter. Add the onion and garlic and cook for 3 minutes. Add the cauliflower rice, remaining ½ tablespoon of Mexican spice blend, remaining 1 teaspoon of salt, and remaining ½ teaspoon of pepper and cook for 15 to 20 minutes until the cauliflower is cooked through, stirring occasionally.

3. To assemble, divide the cauliflower and ground beef evenly among four bowls. Top each bowl with the toppings of your choice.

INGREDIENT TIP: Cauliflower rice is extremely versatile in any dish and that's why I keep several bags in the freezer at all times. You can find it in the frozen section of the grocery store.

PER SERVING (1 bowl without toppings)

Calories: 306; Total Fat: 20g; Protein: 24g; Total Carbs: 7.5g; Fiber: 3g; Net Carbs: 4.5g

ROSEMARY MINT MARINATED LAMB CHOPS

SERVES 4 | PREP TIME: 5 MINUTES, PLUS 30 MINUTES TO MARINATE | COOK TIME: 10 MINUTES

EGG-FREE · NUT-FREE · PALEO/DAIRY-FREE

Tender lamb chops cooked with fresh rosemary and mint are delectable, especially when they are cooked to a perfect medium-rare.

3 tablespoons extra-virgin olive oil, plus more for greasing

½ teaspoon sea salt

1 tablespoon fresh rosemary leaves (from about 4 sprigs), plus more sprigs for garnish

1 tablespoon chopped mint leaves

½ teaspoon garlic salt

4 (4-ounce) lamb chops (about ½-inch thick)

Freshly ground black pepper

1. In a blender, combine the olive oil, salt, rosemary, mint, and garlic salt and blend until smooth. Rub the mixture all over the lamb chops and let them marinate in an airtight container in the refrigerator for 30 minutes or up to 4 hours.

2. Oil a large skillet over medium-high heat. Add the lamb chops and cook for about 3 minutes on each side (for medium-rare), or to desired doneness.

3. Plate the chops and let them rest for 3 minutes. Pour the leftover extra juices over the lamb chops and garnish with rosemary sprigs and pepper.

VARIATION TIP: This marinade also works great on a lamb loin.

PER SERVING (1 chop)

Calories: 254; Total Fat: 18g; Protein: 23g; Total Carbs: 0g; Fiber: 0g; Net Carbs: 0g

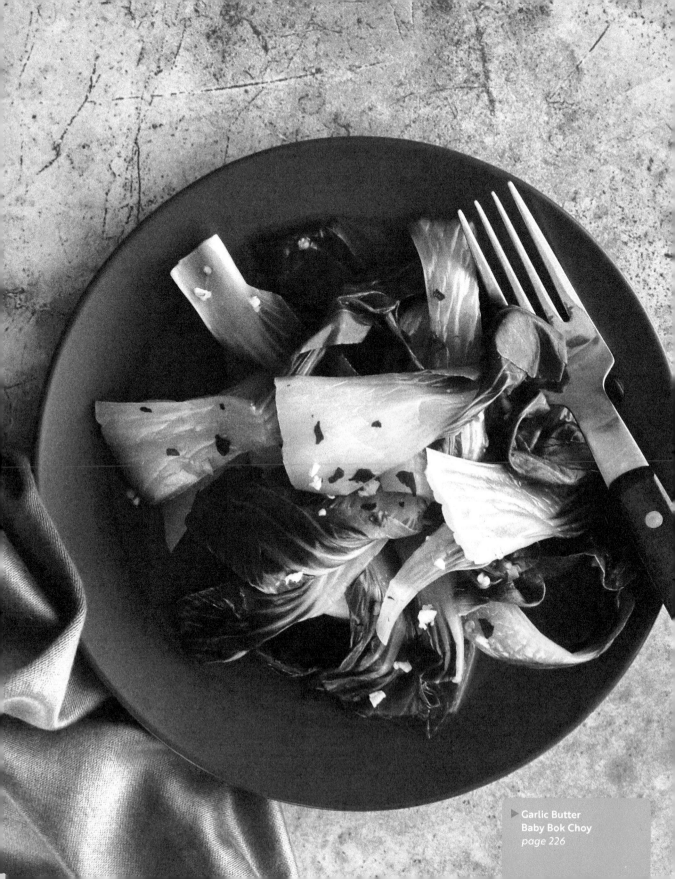

Garlic Butter
Baby Bok Choy
page 226

Vegetables and Sides

SMASHED GUACAMOLE

SERVES 8 | PREP TIME: 10 MINUTES

EGG-FREE · NUT-FREE · PALEO/DAIRY-FREE · VEGAN · BULK PREP

You might be used to seeing guacamole in a big dish all mixed into a purée and served with chips, but that's just not how it goes in keto. Enjoy this more casual version on top of burgers, next to steak, and with your taco salads!

3 ripe avocados

6 cherry tomatoes, roughly chopped

¼ cup roughly chopped fresh cilantro or parsley

⅓ cup finely chopped red onion

1½ tablespoons freshly squeezed lime juice

½ teaspoon sea salt

¼ teaspoon garlic powder

Pinch red pepper flakes

1. In a bowl, combine all of the ingredients and use a fork to mash everything together to your desired consistency.

2. Serve immediately, or store in an airtight container for a few days.

RECIPE TIP: This recipe is particularly good loosely mashed on hamburgers and salads. Avocado is full of great fats, so a small serving is quite filling!

PER SERVING

Calories: 100; Total Fat: 8g; Protein: 1g; Total Carbs: 6g; Fiber: 4g; Net Carbs: 2g

CAULIFLOWER MUSHROOM RISOTTO

SERVES 6 | PREP TIME: 15 MINUTES | COOK TIME: 30 MINUTES

EGG-FREE · NUT-FREE · PALEO/DAIRY-FREE OPTION · VEGETARIAN · BULK PREP

This is one of the very first recipes I made using cauliflower rice. I was blown away by the fact that I could not tell the difference at all from using regular rice. If you let it simmer long enough over low heat, the cauliflower rice absorbs the sauce extremely well and becomes super flavorful. Top with 1 tablespoon of pine nuts for added crunch and serve with your protein of choice for a delicious, hearty meal.

2 tablespoons butter or ghee

½ cup chopped onion

4 garlic cloves, minced

2 teaspoons dried basil

2 teaspoons dried parsley

⅛ teaspoon cayenne pepper (optional)

3 cups (about 8 ounces) chopped baby bella mushrooms

2 cups fresh or frozen cauliflower rice

1 cup Bone Broth (page 240)

1 teaspoon sea salt

1 teaspoon freshly ground black pepper

1 cup freshly grated Parmesan cheese

1. In a large skillet, melt the butter over medium heat. Add the onion, garlic, basil, parsley, and cayenne (if using). Cook, stirring, for 2 minutes. Add the mushrooms and cook for about 5 minutes until the mushrooms begin to soften.

2. Add the cauliflower, bone broth, salt, and pepper and cook, stirring occasionally, for 15 to 20 minutes until the cauliflower and mushrooms have absorbed most of the broth. Add the cheese and stir until melted.

3. Store in the refrigerator for the week for a ready-made side dish, or freeze and defrost the night before serving.

MAKE IT PALEO/DAIRY-FREE: Replace the cheese with ¼ cup full-fat canned coconut milk and a few tablespoons of nutritional yeast.

PER SERVING (about ¾ cup)

Calories: 154; Total Fat: 10g; Protein: 9g; Total Carbs: 7g; Fiber: 2g; Net Carbs: 5g

KETO REFRIED "BEANS"

MAKES 8 CUPS | PREP TIME: 20 MINUTES | COOK TIME: 55 MINUTES

EGG-FREE · NUT-FREE · PALEO/DAIRY-FREE OPTION · VEGETARIAN OPTION · BULK PREP

Beans are high in carbs and therefore not usually part of a ketogenic lifestyle. However, if you're a bean lover, these keto refried "beans" will definitely become a staple in your keto household. The eggplant and zucchini, once cooked and pureed, mimic the texture of mashed beans so well that when I first tasted these, I literally thought I was eating refried beans at a traditional Mexican restaurant, but better!

1 pound bacon

3 eggplants, peeled and chopped

3 zucchini, chopped

1 onion, chopped

1 jalapeño pepper, finely chopped

6 garlic cloves, minced

2 tablespoons ground cumin

1 tablespoon dried oregano

1 tablespoon dried parsley

1 teaspoon chili powder

½ teaspoon cayenne pepper

Sea salt

Freshly ground black pepper

1 cup shredded sharp Cheddar cheese

1. In a large skillet, cook the bacon over medium-high heat in two to three batches, for 5 to 7 minutes each, until crisp. Remove the cooked bacon to a paper towel, leaving the grease in the skillet.

2. Add the eggplant and zucchini to the skillet and cook until soft, about 15 minutes. Using a slotted spoon, transfer the eggplant and zucchini to a food processor, leaving as much bacon grease in the pan as possible. Add the bacon to the food processor and pulse 4 to 5 times until the mixture is smooth.

3. Add the onion, jalapeño, garlic, cumin, oregano, parsley, chili powder, cayenne, salt, and pepper to the skillet. Cook until the onion is soft, 8 to 10 minutes. Add the eggplant mixture to the skillet and stir to combine.

4. Stir in the cheese, reduce the heat to low, and simmer for 10 to 15 minutes.

5. To store, let the mixture cool completely. Using a ½-cup measuring cup, divide the mixture into 16 small freezer-safe plastic bags or mini glass containers. Or, if you're cooking for more than one person, you can use a 1-cup measuring cup and divide into 8 servings (or 4 servings for 4 people). Store in the freezer for up to 3 months. Pull it out whenever you're craving a side of refried beans to go along with your keto-fied meal. Just thaw the night before in the refrigerator and reheat in the oven or microwave.

MAKE IT PALEO/DAIRY-FREE: Leave out the cheese.

MAKE IT VEGETARIAN: Leave out the bacon and use 3 to 4 tablespoons of avocado or coconut oil for sautéing the vegetables.

PER SERVING (½ cup)

Calories: 179; Total Fat: 13g; Protein: 7g; Total Carbs: 8.5g; Fiber: 3.5g; Net Carbs: 5g

GARLIC BUTTER BABY BOK CHOY

SERVES 4 | PREP TIME: 5 MINUTES | COOK TIME: 20 MINUTES

EGG-FREE · NUT-FREE · VEGETARIAN OPTION · UNDER 30 MINUTES

Baby bok choy is slowly becoming one of my new favorite go-to veggies. It's nutrient-dense, very low in carbs, and soaks up any sauce that you pair it with. This recipe calls for a quick sauté, but baby bok choy is also great thrown on the grill or as a colorful and nutritious addition to soups or stews.

3 tablespoons butter or ghee

4 garlic cloves, minced

1½ pounds baby bok choy (about 12 small heads), ends trimmed off and halved lengthwise

1 cup Bone Broth (page 240)

1 teaspoon sea salt

½ teaspoon freshly ground black pepper

½ teaspoon ground ginger

Pinch red pepper flakes

1. In a large skillet over medium heat, melt the butter. Add the garlic and cook until fragrant, 3 to 5 minutes.

2. Add the bok choy to the garlic butter and stir to evenly coat. Add the bone broth, salt, pepper, and ginger. Simmer for 10 to 15 minutes until the bok choy is fork-tender.

3. Sprinkle with red pepper flakes and serve.

MAKE IT VEGETARIAN: Replace the bone broth with vegetable broth.

PER SERVING (6 halves)

Calories: 113; Total Fat: 9g; Protein: 3g; Total Carbs: 5g; Fiber: 2g; Net Carbs: 3g

ZESTY ROASTED BROCCOLI

SERVES 4 | PREP TIME: 5 MINUTES | COOK TIME: 30 MINUTES

EGG-FREE · NUT-FREE · PALEO/DAIRY-FREE OPTION · VEGETARIAN

If you've never tried roasted broccoli before, you're missing out. It has a completely different texture and taste compared to the traditional steamed version. It's one of my favorite side dishes that pairs well with any protein.

4 cups broccoli florets (about 10 ounces)

2 tablespoons melted lard, tallow, coconut oil, or other preferred fat

2 tablespoons freshly squeezed lemon juice

1 teaspoon garlic powder

1 teaspoon sea salt

½ teaspoon freshly ground black pepper

1 teaspoon lemon zest

½ teaspoon red pepper flakes

½ cup freshly grated Parmesan cheese

1. Preheat the oven to 400°F. Line a large baking sheet with parchment paper or a silicone mat.

2. Arrange the broccoli in a single layer on the prepared baking sheet and drizzle with the lard or oil. Toss with your hands so all the pieces are coated.

3. Drizzle the lemon juice on top of the broccoli and then sprinkle with the garlic powder, salt, pepper, lemon zest, and red pepper flakes.

4. Bake for 20 to 25 minutes until fork-tender.

5. Sprinkle with the Parmesan and bake for another 5 minutes or until the cheese is melted.

MAKE IT PALEO/DAIRY-FREE: Substitute nutritional yeast for the Parmesan.

PER SERVING

Calories: 147; Total Fat: 11g; Protein: 7g; Total Carbs: 5g; Fiber: 2g; Net Carbs: 3g

EASY CREAMY MUSHROOMS

SERVES 4 | PREP TIME: 10 MINUTES | COOK TIME: 20 MINUTES

EGG-FREE · NUT-FREE · VEGETARIAN · UNDER 30 MINUTES

A quick and simple recipe that's bursting with flavor, these creamy mushrooms make a perfect topping for grilled steak, pork chops, or even a simple side dish all on their own. Feel free to mix up the spices or add fresh herbs to jazz it up a bit.

2 tablespoons butter or ghee

3 garlic cloves, minced

1 pound mushrooms, sliced (about 6 cups sliced)

1 teaspoon onion powder

1 teaspoon dried oregano

½ teaspoon dried thyme

½ teaspoon sea salt

¼ teaspoon freshly ground black pepper

¼ cup heavy (whipping) cream

½ cup freshly grated Parmesan (or other sharp cheese)

1. In a large skillet over medium heat, melt the butter. Add the garlic and cook for 3 minutes. Add the mushrooms, onion powder, oregano, thyme, salt, and pepper. Cook for 5 minutes, stirring occasionally, until the mushrooms start to soften.

2. Reduce the heat to medium-low and stir in the cream and Parmesan. Bring to a light simmer and cook for about 10 minutes or until the sauce thickens.

VARIATION TIP: Feel free to mix up the spices or use fresh herbs to give this dish another kick.

PER SERVING

Calories: 165; Total Fat: 13g; Protein: 6g; Total Carbs: 6g; Fiber: 2g; Net Carbs: 4g

BACON-WRAPPED ASPARAGUS BUNDLES

SERVES 8 | PREP TIME: 5 MINUTES | COOK TIME: 25 MINUTES

EGG-FREE · NUT-FREE · PALEO/DAIRY-FREE · UNDER 30 MINUTES

With only two main ingredients and a super-fast prep time, this recipe is perfect for those busy nights when you need a quick side dish. Pair these yummy bundles of bacon-wrapped goodness with a juicy steak or roasted chicken thighs for a simple and delicious meal.

1 tablespoon melted coconut oil or other preferred fat, plus additional for greasing

2 pounds asparagus, trimmed

1 teaspoon garlic powder

1 teaspoon sea salt

½ teaspoon freshly ground black pepper

8 bacon slices

1. Preheat the oven to 400°F. Line a rimmed baking sheet with aluminum foil. Place a wire rack over the baking sheet and grease with oil.

2. Lightly coat the asparagus with the oil and then season with the garlic powder, salt, and pepper.

3. Divide the asparagus evenly into 8 bundles. Wrap a slice of bacon around each asparagus bundle, starting at the bottom of the stalks and working upward.

4. Place each bundle on the wire rack and bake for 15 to 20 minutes until the asparagus is fork-tender.

5. Turn the oven to broil and cook for an additional 3 to 5 minutes to allow the bacon to crisp up.

RECIPE TIP: Cooking time may vary depending on the thickness of your asparagus spears.

PER SERVING (1 bundle)

Calories: 100; Total Fat: 6g; Protein: 7g; Total Carbs: 4.5g; Fiber: 2.5g; Net Carbs: 2g

KETO VEGETABLE PAD THAI

SERVES 4 | PREP TIME: 10 MINUTES | COOK TIME: 20 MINUTES

EGG-FREE · PALEO/DAIRY-FREE · UNDER 30 MINUTES

Who doesn't love a big bowl of yummy, flavorful noodles with a slightly sweet, tangy sauce? This is my take on keto-friendly Pad Thai using shirataki noodles. Pair it with your favorite protein and you've got a quick, tasty meal.

FOR THE SAUCE

2 tablespoons peanut butter
   (or almond butter)

2 garlic cloves, minced (or 1 teaspoon garlic powder)

2 tablespoons fish sauce

1 tablespoon coconut aminos

1 tablespoon coconut vinegar
   or apple cider vinegar

1 teaspoon chili paste

¼ teaspoon ground ginger (optional)

Dash sweetener

FOR THE NOODLES

2 tablespoons coconut oil

2 cups chopped broccoli

3 (7-ounce) packages shirataki noodles, rinsed and thoroughly drained

2 cups bean sprouts

2 scallions, chopped

Sea salt

Freshly ground black pepper

½ cup chopped fresh basil (optional)

¼ cup chopped roasted peanuts (optional)

Lime wedges for serving (optional)

TO MAKE THE SAUCE

In a small microwave-safe bowl, heat the peanut butter in the microwave for 20 to 30 seconds until melted. Add the garlic, fish sauce, coconut aminos, vinegar, chili paste, ginger (if using), and sweetener. Whisk to combine, taste, and adjust the sweetness or spiciness depending on your preference.

TO MAKE THE NOODLES

1. In a large wok or skillet, melt the coconut oil over medium-high heat. Add the broccoli and cook, stirring occasionally, for 5 minutes. Add the noodles, bean sprouts, and scallions and pour in the sauce. Toss to mix well and sauté for 10 to 15 minutes until the broccoli is cooked through. Taste and season with salt and pepper.

2. Remove from the heat and toss in the basil (if using). Serve garnished with peanuts and lime wedges (if using).

PER SERVING

Calories: 211; Total Fat: 15g; Protein: 8g; Total Carbs: 11g; Fiber: 5g; Net Carbs: 6g

LOADED CAULIFLOWER "BAKED POTATO" CASSEROLE

SERVES 5 | PREP TIME: 5 MINUTES | COOK TIME: 30 MINUTES

EGG-FREE · NUT-FREE

Credit for this recipe goes to my best friend, Alex. She's been my personal recipe taste tester for a while now, and when she came up with this recipe herself and asked me to try it, I was very impressed. It's simple to make and I promise you won't even miss the potato when you dig into this tasty casserole.

4 bacon slices

4 cups fresh or frozen cauliflower rice

1 teaspoon garlic powder

1 teaspoon onion powder

½ teaspoon chili powder

½ teaspoon sea salt

¼ teaspoon freshly ground black pepper

1 cup shredded Cheddar cheese

5 tablespoons sour cream

1 large scallion, chopped

1. Preheat the oven to 350°F.
2. In a large skillet over medium-high heat, cook the bacon until crisp, 5 to 7 minutes.
3. Once cooked, remove the bacon to a paper towel, leaving the grease in the skillet.
4. Add the cauliflower rice, garlic powder, onion powder, chili powder, salt, and pepper to the skillet. Sauté, stirring occasionally, for about 10 minutes or until the cauliflower starts to soften.
5. Transfer the cauliflower mixture to an 8-by-8-inch baking dish. Crumble the bacon on top and then sprinkle with the Cheddar.
6. Bake for 10 to 12 minutes until the cheese is melted.
7. To serve, top each dish with 1 tablespoon of sour cream and a sprinkle of chopped scallion.

INGREDIENT TIP: Buying frozen cauliflower rice in bulk and dividing it into smaller portions to store in the freezer makes dishes like these very simple and budget-friendly.

PER SERVING (¾ cup)

Calories: 208; Total Fat: 16g; Protein: 9g; Total Carbs: 7g; Fiber: 2g; Net Carbs: 5g

SHEET-PAN GREEN BEAN CASSEROLE

SERVES 6 | PREP TIME: 10 MINUTES | COOK TIME: 20 MINUTES

EGG-FREE · PALEO/DAIRY-FREE · BULK PREP · UNDER 30 MINUTES

All the flavor of a green bean casserole laid out on a baking sheet for all to see. Get green with your beans and full on your fats from a sincerely delicious portion of crispy bacon. Garnish with slivered almonds for extra crunch.

3 cups (about 1 pound) green beans, trimmed

1 (12-ounce) package bacon (about 14 slices), chopped

¼ white onion, cut into thin rings

2 tablespoons extra-virgin olive oil

¼ cup slivered almonds

1 teaspoon garlic powder

1 teaspoon sea salt

1 teaspoon freshly ground black pepper

1. Preheat the oven to 425°F. Line a baking sheet (or two, so that the veggies don't overlap too much) with parchment paper or aluminum foil.

2. In a large bowl, combine the green beans, bacon, onion, oil, almonds, and garlic powder and toss to coat. Spread the mixture out in an even layer on the baking sheet(s). Sprinkle the salt and pepper generously over everything.

3. Bake for about 20 minutes. Serve immediately.

RECIPE TIP: To avoid nut allergies, simply skip the slivered almonds.

PER SERVING

Calories: 199; Total Fat: 15g; Protein: 9g; Total Carbs: 7g; Fiber: 3g; Net Carbs: 4g

SLOW COOKER CREAMED SPINACH AND ARTICHOKE

SERVES 12 | PREP TIME: 10 MINUTES | COOK TIME: 2 TO 3 HOURS ON LOW

EGG-FREE · NUT-FREE · VEGETARIAN · BULK PREP

This side dish pays homage to your traditional spinach and artichoke dip, except it's a heartier, meatier version that holds its own as a side. You can serve this savory side next to steak or chicken.

16 ounces cream cheese

1 tablespoon minced garlic

½ cup freshly grated Parmesan cheese, plus 1 cup shredded

½ teaspoon sea salt

1 teaspoon garlic powder

1 cup marinated artichoke hearts, chopped

12 ounces fresh baby spinach

1. Preheat the slow cooker to low.

2. In a microwave-safe bowl, microwave the cream cheese for about 1 minute. Transfer it to the slow cooker. Stir in the garlic, ½ cup of grated Parmesan, salt, garlic powder, artichokes, and spinach. Sprinkle the remaining 1 cup of shredded Parmesan cheese over the top.

3. Cook on low for 2 to 3 hours.

4. Serve immediately or refrigerate for up to 5 days in an airtight container.

VARIATION TIP: For a blast of color, substitute roasted red peppers for the artichokes.

PER SERVING

Calories: 193; Total Fat: 17g; Protein: 6g; Total Carbs: 4g; Fiber: 1g; Net Carbs: 3g

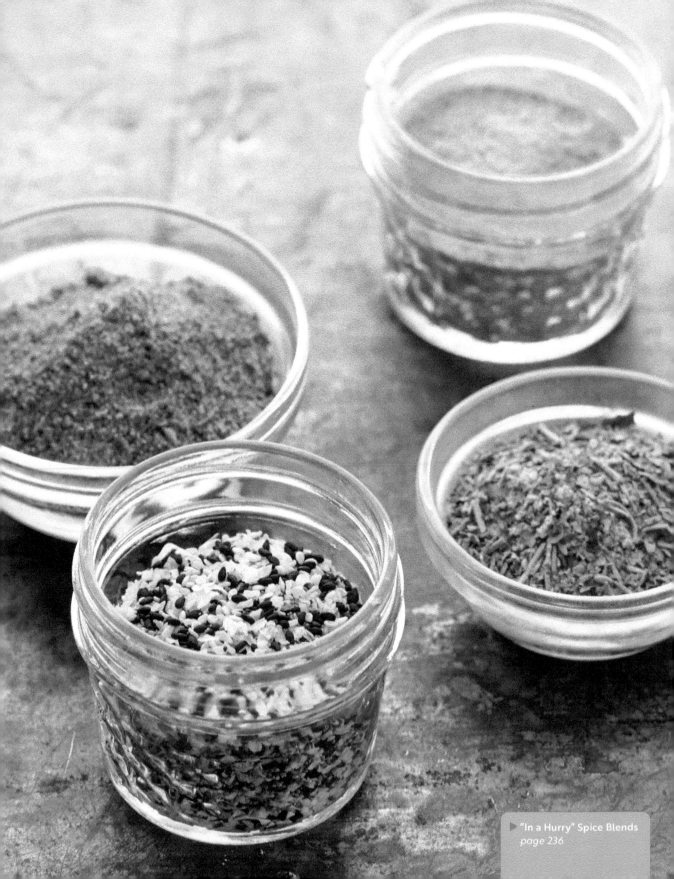

▶ "In a Hurry" Spice Blends
page 236

12

Staples

"IN A HURRY" SPICE BLENDS

PREP TIME: 5 MINUTES

EGG-FREE · NUT-FREE · PALEO/DAIRY-FREE · BULK PREP · UNDER 30 MINUTES

Having these blends ready to go makes cooking easy and adds flavor to any dish. Use 4-ounce baby food jars to store the different blends, or any airtight container. If you cook a lot, double or triple the blends so you have them on hand. Store them in a cool dry place and shake well before using.

Everything Seasoning

MAKES 5 TABLESPOONS

1 tablespoon sesame seeds

1 tablespoon poppy seeds

1 tablespoon black sesame seeds

2 teaspoons dried minced garlic

2 teaspoons dried minced onion

2 teaspoons sea salt flakes

Combine all the ingredients in an airtight container, shake well, and store at room temperature.

RECIPE TIP: Toast the sesame seeds for a nuttier flavor.

PER SERVING (1 tablespoon)

Calories: 35; Total Fat: 2.5g; Protein: 1g; Total Carbs: 2g; Fiber: 1g; Net Carbs: 1g

Indian Spice Blend

MAKES 5 TABLESPOONS

1 tablespoon garam masala

1 tablespoon ground turmeric

2 teaspoons onion powder

2 teaspoons garlic powder

1 teaspoon ground ginger

1 teaspoon ground cumin

1 teaspoon sea salt

½ teaspoon freshly ground
   black pepper

Combine all the ingredients in an airtight container, shake well, and store at room temperature.

PER SERVING (1 tablespoon)

Calories: 20; Total Fat: 0g; Protein: 1g; Total Carbs: 4g; Fiber: 1.5g; Net Carbs: 2.5g

Mediterranean Spice Blend

MAKES 5 TABLESPOONS

1 tablespoon dried oregano

1 tablespoon dried rosemary

1 tablespoon dried parsley

2 teaspoons garlic powder

1 teaspoon onion powder

1 teaspoon lemon-pepper seasoning

1 teaspoon dried basil

1 teaspoon sea salt

¼ teaspoon red pepper flakes
(optional)

Combine all the ingredients in an airtight container, shake well, and store at room temperature.

RECIPE TIP: Muddle or crush the rosemary to break it up into smaller pieces for the blend.

PER SERVING (1 tablespoon)

Calories: 12; Total Fat: 0g; Protein: 0.5g; Total Carbs: 2.5g; Fiber: 1g; Net Carbs: 1.5g

Mexican Spice Blend

MAKES 5 TABLESPOONS

2 tablespoons chili powder

1 tablespoon ground cumin

2 teaspoons onion powder

2 teaspoons garlic powder

1 teaspoon ground coriander

1 teaspoon paprika

1 teaspoon dried oregano

1 teaspoon sea salt

½ teaspoon freshly ground
black pepper

⅛ teaspoon cayenne pepper

Combine all the ingredients in an airtight container, shake well, and store at room temperature.

PER SERVING (1 tablespoon)

Calories: 29; Total Fat: 1g; Protein: 1g; Total Carbs: 4g; Fiber: 2g; Net Carbs: 2g

FAT-BURNING DRESSING

MAKES ABOUT ½ CUP | PREP TIME: 5 MINUTES

NUT-FREE · PALEO/DAIRY-FREE · BULK PREP · UNDER 30 MINUTES

Most store-bought salad dressings are made with unhealthy oils like canola, sunflower, and safflower oil. These oils are very inflammatory to your body, and even though they may be low in carbs, they are still not ideal. This Fat-Burning Dressing is quick and easy to make and can be flavored with the spices and herbs of your choice. Make sure to use avocado- or olive oil–based mayonnaise for the reasons I mentioned.

¼ cup mayonnaise

¼ cup MCT oil

2 garlic cloves

2 teaspoons apple cider vinegar or coconut vinegar

2 teaspoons Dijon mustard

1 teaspoon your choice "In a Hurry" Spice Blend (page 236) or choice of fresh herbs

½ teaspoon sea salt

¼ teaspoon freshly ground black pepper

1. In a medium bowl or in a blender, combine the mayonnaise, MCT oil, garlic, vinegar, mustard, spice blend, salt, and pepper and purée (use an immersion blender to purée in the bowl) until smooth.

2. Store in an airtight container in the refrigerator for up to 3 weeks.

INGREDIENT TIP: I love using MCT oil to make dressings because it has a neutral flavor so you can make virtually any dressing with it. If you don't have MCT oil, you could use avocado or olive oil.

RECIPE TIP: The oil may separate a bit while sitting in the refrigerator. Simply shake or stir it up when ready to serve.

PER SERVING (1 tablespoon)

Calories: 101; Total Fat: 11g; Protein: 0g; Total Carbs: 0.5g; Fiber: 0g; Net Carbs: 0.5g

ZESTY PARMESAN ITALIAN DRESSING

MAKES 2 CUPS | PREP TIME: 10 MINUTES, PLUS 1 HOUR TO REST

EGG-FREE · **NUT-FREE** · **PALEO** · **VEGETARIAN** · **BULK PREP**

Italians don't pre-mix their dressing, so anything made in advance is an American tradition, not an Italian one. This recipe was brought over from Italy by the daughter of Italian immigrants who married the owner of a café that eventually became Ken's Steak House in Framingham, Massachusetts. Sound familiar? This recipe is a bit fancier than the original, but certainly owes all of its flavor to Ken's leading lady.

1 cup extra-virgin olive oil

½ cup white vinegar

1 tablespoon red wine vinegar

2 tablespoons water

2 tablespoons freshly grated Parmesan cheese

1 tablespoon minced garlic

1 tablespoon minced shallots

1 teaspoon dried basil

½ teaspoon dried oregano

¼ teaspoon sea salt

¼ teaspoon freshly ground black pepper

⅛ teaspoon dried marjoram

Pinch red pepper flakes

1. In an airtight container, combine the oil and vinegars and shake. Add the rest of the ingredients and shake again.

2. Let sit on the counter for at least 1 hour before serving, for the flavors to mix.

3. Refrigerate for up to 1 week, allowing 20 minutes before serving to bring to room temperature, and shake again.

VARIATION TIP: If you want less "zest," simply nix the red pepper flakes.

INGREDIENT TIP: Be mindful when purchasing olive oil from your grocery store because there are some brands that mix the olive oil with canola or other vegetable oils because it's cheaper for them. Research the brand of olive oil you are purchasing and make sure it is sold in a dark bottle to prevent rancidity.

PER SERVING (2 tablespoons)

Calories: 119; Total Fat: 13g; Protein: 0.3g; Total Carbs: 0.3g; Fiber: 0.1g; Net Carbs: 0.2g

BONE BROTH

MAKES 4 QUARTS | PREP TIME: 10 MINUTES | COOK TIME: 24 TO 48 HOURS

EGG-FREE · NUT-FREE · PALEO/DAIRY-FREE · BULK PREP

Bone broth is one of the most nutrient-dense foods/drinks that you can consume. It's rich in vitamins and minerals and is amazing for supporting bones, joints, skin, and gut health. I always cook a big batch and store it in individual containers in the freezer. When a recipe calls for bone broth, just thaw one container in the refrigerator overnight the night before and you're good to go.

3 celery stalks, roughly chopped

1 medium onion, cut into quarters

4 garlic cloves, smashed

4 or 5 large beef bones (about 4 pounds) or 1 whole chicken or fish carcass (with skin)

1 bunch fresh rosemary, parsley, or other herbs of choice

1 tablespoon sea salt

1 tablespoon whole peppercorns

2 tablespoons apple cider vinegar or coconut vinegar

1. Preheat the oven to 375°F.

2. In a large roasting pan or baking sheet, arrange the celery, onion, and garlic in an even layer. Place the bones on top of the vegetables and roast in the oven for 30 minutes.

3. Remove the bones and vegetables from the oven and transfer to a slow cooker. Add the fresh herbs, salt, peppercorns, and vinegar. Add enough water to cover the bones and vegetables, at least 4 quarts.

4. Cover and cook on low for 24 to 48 hours. The longer the broth cooks, the more nutrients will be extracted from the bones.

5. Let the broth cool completely, strain it, and then store it in glass containers with airtight lids in the refrigerator or freezer. Make sure to only fill the containers three-quarters full, to allow room for the liquid to expand in the freezer and prevent containers from cracking.

RECIPE TIP: Add chicken feet and fish heads to boost the collagen and flavor of your bone broth.

PER SERVING (1 cup)

Calories: 65; Total Fat: 5g; Protein: 4g; Total Carbs: 1g; Fiber: 0g; Net Carbs: 1g

EASY KETO BREAD

SERVES 12 | PREP TIME: 10 MINUTES | COOK TIME: 45 MINUTES

PALEO/DAIRY-FREE OPTION · VEGETARIAN · BULK PREP

Who says you can't have bread on a ketogenic diet? This keto bread is a staple in my house and is extremely versatile for use in several different recipes. You can flavor it however you'd like with seeds and spices. It stores perfectly in the freezer for months at a time. I divide my loaf into four portions, keep one in the refrigerator for the week and freeze the rest in separate freezer-safe containers or bags.

Butter or coconut oil, for greasing

9 eggs, at room temperature

6 tablespoons butter or ghee, melted and cooled

2¼ cups almond flour

1 tablespoon baking powder

1 teaspoon sea salt

1. Preheat the oven to 350°F. Grease a 9-by-5 inch loaf pan with butter or coconut oil and line it with parchment paper.

2. In a large bowl or stand mixer, beat the eggs on high for 2 minutes. The eggs will get fluffy and bubbles will form.

3. With the mixer on low speed, add the cooled melted butter into the eggs in a slow stream.

4. In a separate bowl, whisk together the almond flour, baking powder, and salt using a fork.

5. Slowly add the almond flour mixture to the eggs, one-quarter of the mixture at a time. Mix with the fork after each addition until well combined.

6. Pour the mixture into the prepared pan and bake for 35 to 45 minutes until golden brown on top and a toothpick inserted in the center comes out clean.

7. Let cool on a baking rack.

8. Store in the refrigerator for up to 1 week or slice and freeze for up to 3 months.

INGREDIENT TIP: If you don't have baking powder, you can use 1 teaspoon baking soda plus 2 teaspoons cream of tartar as a replacement for 1 tablespoon baking powder.

MAKE IT PALEO/DAIRY-FREE: Replace the butter or ghee with olive oil or coconut oil

PER SERVING (1 slice)

Calories: 236; Total Fat: 20g; Protein: 9g; Total Carbs: 5g; Fiber: 2.5g; Net Carbs: 2.5g.

KETO DOUGH THREE WAYS

NUT-FREE OPTION · PALEO/DAIRY-FREE OPTION · BULK PREP · UNDER 30 MINUTES

Pizza, crackers, flat breads, pot pies—these are just some of the many ways you can use these keto-friendly doughs. They are simple to make, can be flavored however you like, and you can even make a few batches at a time and store them in the freezer. Thaw them in the refrigerator overnight the night before and you're good to go! See below for recipes that use keto dough in this book and experiment with these doughs to replace traditional dough in other recipes like empanadas or calzones.

Traditional Keto Dough

1½ cups (about 6 ounces) shredded mozzarella cheese

2 tablespoons cream cheese

¾ cup almond flour

Seasonings of choice

1 egg

PER BATCH OF TRADITIONAL KETO DOUGH

Calories: 1,199; Total Fat: 95g; Protein: 64g; Total Carbs: 22g; Fiber: 9g; Net Carbs: 13g

1. Put the mozzarella and cream cheese in a microwave-safe bowl. Microwave for 45 seconds and then stir until combined. If the cheese isn't completely melted, microwave for another 10 to 15 seconds.

2. Meanwhile, in a small bowl, whisk together the almond flour and seasonings of choice.

3. Add the almond flour mixture to the cheese along with the egg. Knead, starting with a spatula and then using your hands (if desired) until the dough comes together. If the dough becomes hard to mix, microwave for another 10 to 15 seconds to soften.

Paleo/Dairy-Free Keto Dough

1 cup almond flour

1 cup crushed pork rinds (or substitute another ½ cup almond flour)

Seasonings of choice

2 eggs

1 tablespoon avocado oil or coconut oil

PER BATCH OF PALEO/DAIRY-FREE KETO DOUGH

Calories: 1,284; Total Fat: 100g; Protein: 72g; Total Carbs: 24g; Fiber: 12g; Net Carbs: 12g

1. In a medium bowl, mix together the almond flour, pork rinds, and seasonings of choice.

2. Add the eggs and oil and then knead, starting with a spatula and then using your hands (if desired) until the dough comes together.

Nut-Free Keto Dough

1½ cups (about 6 ounces) shredded mozzarella cheese

2 tablespoons cream cheese

⅓ cup coconut flour

Seasonings of choice

1 egg

PER BATCH OF NUT-FREE KETO DOUGH

Calories: 835; Total Fat: 58g; Protein: 51g; Total Carbs: 25g; Fiber: 13g; Net Carbs: 12g

1. Put the mozzarella and cream cheese in a microwave-safe bowl. Microwave for 45 seconds and then stir until combined. If the cheese is not completely melted, microwave for another 10 to 15 seconds.

2. Meanwhile, in a small bowl, whisk together the coconut flour and seasonings of choice.

CONTINUED

KETO DOUGH THREE WAYS CONTINUED

3. Add the coconut flour mixture to the cheese, along with the egg. Knead, starting with a spatula and then using your hands (if desired) until the dough comes together. If the dough becomes hard to mix, microwave for another 10 to 15 seconds to soften.

RECIPE TIP: If any of the doughs are still sticky and not coming together after combining all of the ingredients, add another teaspoon or two of flour and work it in until the dough is no longer sticky. Different brands and textures of almond and coconut flours may be more or less dry than others.

RECIPES WITH KETO DOUGH:
- Buffalo Chicken Pizza (page 178)
- Keto Crackers (page 136)
- Pizza Bagel Bites (page 137)
- Turkey Pot Pie (page 184)

EASY PEASY GARLICKY PESTO

MAKES 1 CUP | PREP TIME: 5 MINUTES

EGG-FREE · PALEO · VEGETARIAN · BULK PREP · UNDER 30 MINUTES

Despite the name, this pesto doesn't have peas in it, but it *is* easy! Keeping a basil plant in your kitchen is one easy way to make sure you have basil all year long in any climate. They do drink a lot of water and love the sun, though, so make sure you have a plant-sitter to accommodate your ultimate source of all-season pesto!

2 cups (packed) fresh basil leaves

½ cup pine nuts

½ cup freshly grated Parmesan cheese

4 garlic cloves

½ cup extra-virgin olive oil

Pinch ground nutmeg

Sea salt

Freshly ground pepper

1. In a food processor, combine all of the ingredients. Process until smooth.
2. Store in an airtight container to keep the pesto green for a few days, or freeze it for up to 1 month.

VARIATION TIP: For a more peppery flavor, substitute 1 cup of arugula for 1 cup of the basil. You can also substitute pumpkin seeds for the pine nuts. If you love the taste of truffles, another fun twist is adding ½ teaspoon of truffle oil.

PER SERVING (2 tablespoons)

Calories: 200; Total Fat: 20g; Protein: 3g; Total Carbs: 2g; Fiber: 0.5g; Net Carbs: 1.5g

HOMEMADE HAZELNUT BUTTER

MAKES ABOUT 1½ CUPS | PREP TIME: 5 MINUTES, PLUS 20 MINUTES FOR ROASTING

EGG-FREE · PALEO/DAIRY-FREE · VEGAN · BULK PREP · UNDER 30 MINUTES

Tired of searching through the grocery store for a "natural" nut butter that doesn't break the bank? Well, you're in luck! This fast and easy hazelnut butter recipe can be made with any type of nut or seed of your choice and stores for weeks in the refrigerator. It's delicious, and making it yourself allows you to control both the salt and flavor outcome.

2 cups raw hazelnuts

1½ teaspoons sea salt

½ teaspoon ground cinnamon (optional)

2 tablespoons MCT oil or coconut oil

1. Preheat the oven to 275°F.
2. Pour the hazelnuts onto a baking sheet and roast in the oven for 15 to 20 minutes until golden brown.
3. Combine the hazelnuts, salt, and cinnamon (if using) in a food processor or blender. Pulse a few times and then drizzle in the oil and pulse until smooth.
4. Transfer to a glass jar with an airtight lid and store in the refrigerator.

SUBSTITUTION TIP: Replace the hazelnuts with low-carb nuts of your choice: pili nuts, macadamia nuts, pecans, walnuts, almonds, or peanuts.

PER SERVING (1 tablespoon)

Calories: 97; Total Fat: 9g; Protein: 2g; Total Carbs: 2g; Fiber: 1g; Net Carbs: 1g

MINI FAT BOMBS

MAKES 60 FAT BOMBS | PREP TIME: 5 MINUTES PLUS 1 HOUR TO CHILL

EGG-FREE ° NUT-FREE ° VEGETARIAN ° BULK PREP

These mini fat bombs are perfect for when you're craving a little sweetness. I make a big batch and store them in the freezer for a pre-workout snack or after dinner treat. They're so simple to prepare and because they are "mini," you can enjoy a couple at a time without worrying about going over your calorie or carb goal.

½ cup coconut or MCT oil

½ cup butter or ghee

2 tablespoons unsweetened cacao or cocoa powder

Dash sweetener

Pinch sea salt

1. In a microwave-safe cup or bowl (preferably with a spout) combine the oil, butter, and cacao powder. Microwave for 20 seconds, stir, and then microwave in 10-second increments until melted.

2. Add sweetener and season with salt.

3. Pour the mixture into mini chocolate molds or ice cube trays, about ½ tablespoon per mold.

4. Freeze for at least 1 hour and then pop out of the molds and store in a freezer-safe resealable plastic bag in the freezer.

SPECIAL EQUIPMENT: Mini silicone chocolate molds or ice cube trays.

PER SERVING (2 fat bombs)

Calories: 63; Total Fat: 7g; Protein: 0g; Total Carbs: 0g; Fiber: 0g; Net Carbs: 0g

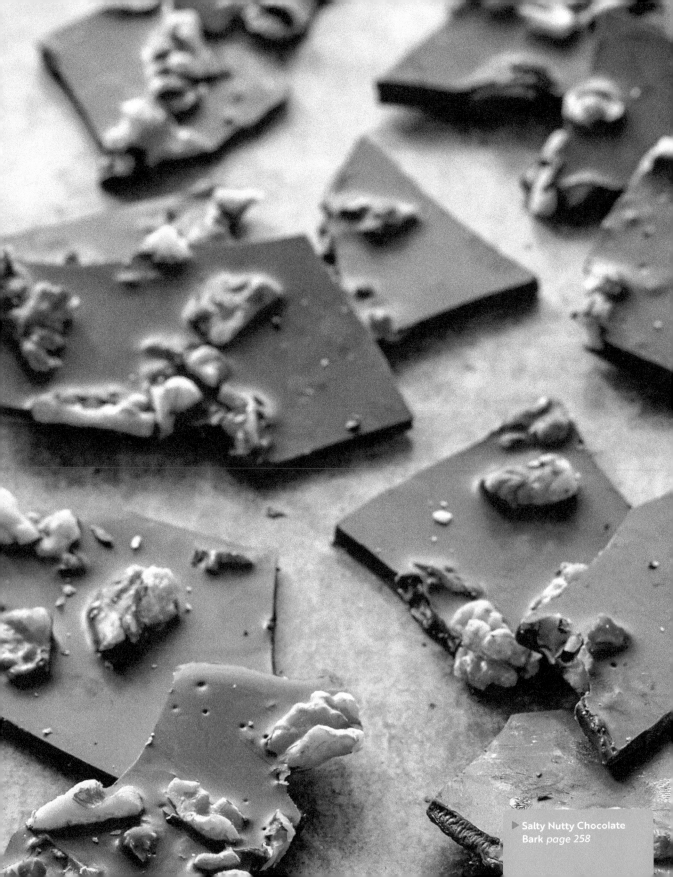

▶ **Salty Nutty Chocolate Bark** *page 258*

13

Sweets

TRAIL MIX WITH DRIED COCONUT AND STRAWBERRIES

MAKES 7 CUPS | PREP TIME: 15 MINUTES | COOK TIME: 3 HOURS 30 MINUTES

EGG-FREE · PALEO/DAIRY-FREE · VEGAN · BULK PREP

This trail mix is great to make for easy snacking or eating with almond milk as cereal for breakfast. The better strawberries you buy, the better they'll be. Peak strawberry season is April through June, so that's a great time to buy and dry your strawberries. I'm also a big fan of buying organic, not just for the hipster cred but because they really do taste sweeter than their watery counterparts.

10 medium strawberries, hulled and halved

2 tablespoons coconut oil

1 teaspoon ground cinnamon

½ teaspoon vanilla extract

Sweetener of choice (optional)

2 cups chopped pecans

2 cups walnut halves, chopped

1 cup unsweetened coconut flakes

½ cup macadamia nuts

½ cup sliced almonds

3 Brazil nuts, chopped

3 tablespoons hulled pumpkin seeds

1. Preheat the oven to 200°F. Line a baking sheet with parchment paper.

2. Arrange the strawberries cut-side up on the prepared baking sheet and bake for 3 hours, rotating the baking sheet every hour. Remove from the oven and let cool for 30 minutes. If they are still moist, cook for another 30 minutes.

3. While the strawberries are cooling, increase the oven heat to 375°F.

4. In a microwave-safe bowl, melt the coconut oil in the microwave. Stir in the cinnamon, vanilla, and sweetener (if using). In another bowl, combine the pecans, walnuts, coconut flakes, macadamia nuts, almonds, Brazil nuts, and pumpkin seeds. Drizzle the coconut oil mixture over the nuts until everything is lightly coated but not soaked.

5. Line two more baking sheets with parchment paper and spread the nut mixture over the sheets evenly. Bake for 15 to 30 minutes until the nuts begin to brown. Remove from the oven and pour onto a paper towel to dry.

6. Once all the ingredients have cooled, toss the nuts and strawberries together and eat right away.

7. If not eating right away, store the strawberries and nuts separately. Both will store safely in an airtight container for 1 week. If moisture develops in your strawberry container, bake for another 30 minutes at 200°F.

VARIATION TIP: You can use any nuts you like, but this recipe uses the nuts with the lowest carbohydrates and highest beneficial fats. If you use others, your nutrition facts may vary. Other lower-carb nuts include pili nuts, hazelnuts, peanuts, pine nuts, and almonds.

PER SERVING (½ cup)

Calories: 388; Total Fat: 36g; Protein: 7g; Total Carbs: 9g; Fiber: 5g; Net Carbs: 4g

FRESH CREAM–FILLED STRAWBERRIES

SERVES 6 | PREP TIME: 10 MINUTES

EGG-FREE · NUT-FREE · VEGETARIAN · UNDER 30 MINUTES

Cream-filled strawberries are some of the simplest desserts you can make, and they're great when you're craving something a little sweet. The high fat content in the heavy cream will satiate your hunger, while the naturally low-sugar strawberries provide a little blast of antioxidants.

1 cup heavy (whipping) cream

Sweetener of choice (optional)

12 large strawberries, hulled and hollowed out

1. In a large bowl, whisk the cream and sweetener (if using) until thickened into whipped cream, about 5 minutes.

2. Spoon the whipped cream into the hollowed strawberries or use a pastry tube to pipe it inside. Serve immediately.

3. Optional garnishes could include lime zest, finely chopped mint, or shaved dark chocolate.

VARIATION TIP: If you plan to serve these at a gathering and they need a longer shelf life, add 3 tablespoons of cream cheese to your cream mixture and increase the sweetener to your desired sweetness. You can also whip the cream faster by using an electric mixer or pouring it into a self serve-size blender for a few seconds.

PER SERVING (2 cream-filled strawberries)

Calories: 153; Total Fat: 15g; Protein: 1g; Total Carbs: 3.5g; Fiber: 0.5g; Net Carbs: 3g

KETO "RICE" PUDDING

SERVES 2 | PREP TIME: 5 MINUTES | COOK TIME: 7 MINUTES

EGG-FREE · NUT-FREE · PALEO/DAIRY-FREE · UNDER 30 MINUTES

This is one of my favorite desserts when I'm looking for volume and want to feel that "fullness" without extra calories and carbs. Shirataki rice is made from the konjac plant, traditionally used in Japanese cuisine and Chinese medicine. The rice is 97 percent water and 3 percent soluble fiber. It's filling due to the high water and fiber content and absorbs the flavors of any dish you pair it with. When you first open the package, you'll notice it has an off-putting smell, but don't worry, the smell goes away once you drain and rinse it. I use the Miracle Noodles brand and pair it with Perfect Keto's Chocolate MCT Powder for a delicious dessert. Shout-out to my good friends Robert Sikes and Danny Vega for this awesome idea!

1 (8-ounce) bag shirataki rice, thoroughly rinsed and drained

1 scoop flavored MCT powder or collagen powder

Pinch Himalayan sea salt

Pinch ground cinnamon

TOPPING SUGGESTIONS

1 tablespoon homemade whipped cream (instruction on page 252)

1 tablespoon chopped nuts (pili nuts, macadamia nuts, walnuts, pecans, almonds)

1 tablespoon chopped dark chocolate or stevia-sweetened chocolate chips

1 tablespoon sugar-free syrup

1. In a small saucepan, bring 1 cup of water to a boil. When the water begins to boil, add the shirataki rice and cook for 2 minutes. Drain in a colander and return to the saucepan.

2. Let any remaining water evaporate and then reduce the heat to medium. Add the MCT powder, salt, and cinnamon. Stir well and cook for another 3 to 5 minutes.

3. Pour into a bowl and add your desired toppings.

RECIPE TIP: Double or triple the recipe and divide into small, airtight containers and store in the refrigerator for the week. When ready to eat, microwave for 30 to 60 seconds, add toppings, and enjoy.

PER SERVING (½ recipe without toppings)

Calories: 58; Total Fat: 4g; Protein: 1g; Total Carbs: 4.5g; Fiber: 4.5g; Net Carbs: 0g

ELECTROLYTE GUMMIES

MAKES 10 GUMMIES | PREP TIME: 5 MINUTES PLUS 30 MINUTES TO CHILL

EGG-FREE · NUT-FREE · PALEO/DAIRY-FREE OPTION · BULK PREP

Gummies that are actually good for you? Yup! Not many people realize it, but gelatin has a ton of health benefits such as joint repair, blood sugar balance, gut health, healthy hair and nails, and more. But it's very important to use a good source of gelatin so you're truly getting all of the benefits (see Ingredient Tip on page 157 for the brands I recommend). In addition to all the benefits from gelatin, these gummies provide you with electrolytes that are essential for maintaining a healthy and successful keto lifestyle. You can buy inexpensive silicone molds on Amazon. If you don't have silicone molds, you can pour the mixture into a glass dish and pop it in the refrigerator to set. Then just cut into squares.

1 cup cold water

2 tablespoons unflavored gelatin

2 packets/scoops flavored electrolyte powder (see Ingredient Tip)

STOVETOP DIRECTIONS

1. In a small saucepan, whisk together the water and gelatin until dissolved. Heat over medium heat for about 5 minutes until it just begins to simmer. Add your flavoring of choice and whisk until well combined.

2. Pour the mixture into silicone molds and refrigerate for 30 to 40 minutes or until set.

3. Pop the gummies out of the molds and enjoy!

MICROWAVE DIRECTIONS

1. Pour the water into a small microwavable bowl or measuring cup (preferably with a spout).
2. Whisk in the gelatin until dissolved and then microwave for 2 minutes or until just starting to bubble.
3. Add your flavoring of choice and whisk until well combined.
4. Pour the mixture into silicone molds and refrigerate for 30 to 40 minutes or until set.
5. Pop the gummies out of the molds and enjoy! Store in an airtight container in the refrigerator for up to 3 weeks.

INGREDIENT TIP: I recommend the Ultima Replenisher Electrolyte Powder brand because it has clean ingredients, zero calories, zero sugar, and is made with plant-based colors and flavors. Plus, all the flavors are delicious and it's packed with tons of vitamins and minerals.

VARIATION TIP: Make a jiggly gelatin desert instead of gummies by using only ½ tablespoon of gelatin. Follow the same directions for the gummies but instead of using molds, pour the mixture into individual containers.

NOTE: Serving size and nutrition facts depend on the size of the molds you are using. I filled my molds with 2 tablespoons each of the mixture to yield 10 servings.

PER SERVING (1 gummy)

Calories: 4; Total Fat: 0g; Protein: 1g; Total Carbs: 0g; Fiber: 0g; Net Carbs: 0g

KETO SNOW CONE

SERVES 1 | PREP TIME: 5 MINUTES

EGG-FREE · NUT-FREE · PALEO/DAIRY-FREE · UNDER 30 MINUTES

This is a great way to satisfy the need for something to munch on while watching your favorite TV show after a long day. It's virtually calorie-free while still satisfying that sweet tooth or late night craving that many of us struggle with.

FOR THE BASE

2 cups ice

FOR SWEET FLAVORS

1 scoop MCT powder or collagen powder (I like the Perfect Keto chocolate or vanilla MCT Powder or Keto Collagen Powder)

1 tablespoon sugar-free syrup

FOR FRUITY FLAVORS

1 packet or scoop of your favorite electrolyte or water enhancer powder (I like the Ultima Replenisher brand)

A few drops of your favorite liquid water enhancer (like Stur or Mio)

Any other zero-calorie liquid or powder flavoring of your choice (sweetened with stevia or monk fruit is preferred)

Crush the ice in a blender. Pour the ice into a shaker bottle and add your flavoring of choice. Cover tightly with a lid and shake well until incorporated. Eat with a spoon.

VARIATION TIP: You could turn this into a milkshake by adding ½ to 1 cup of unsweetened nut/seed milk (coconut, macadamia, hemp, almond) and ½ teaspoon xanthan or guar gum and blending it well.

RECIPE TIP: If you have a Sonic in your area, you can ask for a plain snow cone and flavor it yourself!

NOTE: Nutrition information depends on your add-in of choice.

FIVE-MINUTE KETO COOKIE DOUGH

MAKES 20 DOUGH BALLS | PREP TIME: 5 MINUTES PLUS 1 HOUR TO CHILL

EGG-FREE · NUT-FREE OPTION · BULK PREP

Who doesn't love a big spoonful of chocolate chip cookie dough? This keto cookie dough recipe will bring back those childhood memories without any worry about all the sugar and raw eggs. It won't bake like a regular cookie, but just one bite will knock those sugar cravings out the window.

8 ounces cream cheese, at room temperature

6 tablespoons butter or ghee, at room temperature

½ cup peanut butter (or almond butter)

¼ cup granulated sweetener (such as erythritol)

½ teaspoon vanilla extract

½ to 1 teaspoon monk fruit or stevia, or more (optional)

¼ teaspoon sea salt

¼ cup stevia-sweetened chocolate chips (or >90% dark chocolate chunks)

1. In a large bowl, mix together the cream cheese and butter using an electric hand mixer.

2. Add the peanut butter, granulated sweetener, vanilla, monk fruit, and salt and mix again until well combined. Taste and adjust the sweetness to your liking.

3. Fold in the chocolate chips and then use a tablespoon or small scoop to form 20 dough balls. Arrange the dough balls on a plate or baking sheet.

4. Let chill in the refrigerator for 1 hour and store in an airtight container for up to 3 weeks.

MAKE IT NUT-FREE: You can substitute ¼ cup of coconut flour for the peanut butter or use coconut butter instead.

VARIATION TIP: Add chopped nuts, seeds, unsweetened coconut, or flavored MCT or protein powder to jazz up the cookie dough even more.

PER SERVING (1 dough ball)

Calories: 123; Total Fat: 11g; Protein: 2g; Total Carbs: 4g; Fiber: 1.5g; Net Carbs: 2.5g

SALTY NUTTY CHOCOLATE BARK

MAKES 20 PIECES | PREP TIME: 5 MINUTES PLUS 30 MINUTES TO CHILL | COOK TIME: 10 MINUTES

EGG-FREE · NUT-FREE OPTION · PALEO/DAIRY-FREE · BULK PREP

Chocolate bark is one of the recipes I always make around the holidays because it's so simple and you can jazz it up with whatever toppings you like. You are definitely going to want to add a bit of sweetener because 100 percent chocolate is pretty bitter. I use a few dashes of pure monk fruit or liquid stevia.

½ cup chopped nuts of choice (pecans, pili nuts, macadamia nuts, walnuts, almonds)

8 ounces unsweetened 100 percent dark chocolate

2 tablespoons coconut oil, ghee, or butter

½ to 1 teaspoon sweetener of choice, or more

½ teaspoon sea salt

1. Preheat the oven to 350°F. Line a baking sheet with parchment paper or a silicone mat.

2. Spread the nuts on the prepared baking sheet and toast in the oven for 6 to 8 minutes. Remove from the oven and let cool.

3. Meanwhile, in a microwave-safe dish, mix the chocolate and coconut oil. Microwave in 15-second increments until melted. Add the sweetener and adjust sweetness to your liking.

4. Add the nuts to the chocolate mixture and stir until combined, leaving the parchment paper or silicone mat on the baking sheet.

5. Pour the chocolate mixture onto the baking sheet and spread it out evenly using a spatula. Sprinkle with the sea salt and freeze for 20 to 30 minutes until set.

6. Once set, break the bark into pieces and serve.

7. Store in a resealable plastic bag or airtight container in the freezer.

INGREDIENT TIP: To lower the carb count for this bark, you can swap the unsweetened chocolate with unsweetened cacao butter and a tablespoon of unsweetened cacao/cocoa powder.

MAKE IT NUT-FREE: Replace the nuts with seeds or unsweetened coconut flakes.

PER SERVING (1 piece without nuts)

Calories: 88; Total Fat: 8g; Protein: 2g; Total Carbs: 4g; Fiber: 2g; Net Carbs: 2g

PER SERVING (1 piece with pecans)

Calories: 116; Total Fat: 10g; Protein: 2g; Total Carbs: 4.5g; Fiber: 2g; Net Carbs: 2.5g

NUT BUTTER CUPS

MAKES 12 NUT BUTTER CUPS | PREP TIME: 5 MINUTES, PLUS 40 MINUTES TO CHILL

EGG-FREE · PALEO/DAIRY-FREE · VEGAN · BULK PREP

These nut butter cups are one of my go-to fat bombs. They are super simple to make and easily store in the freezer for a quick dessert or when the urge for chocolate hits. Use your favorite nut butter (preferably homemade) and you've got yourself a keto-friendly treat that's easy and satisfying.

4 ounces unsweetened cacao/cocoa butter, chopped

¼ cup coconut oil, ghee, or butter

2 tablespoons unsweetened cacao/cocoa powder

½ to 1 teaspoon sweetener of choice, or more

6 tablespoons Homemade Hazelnut Butter (page 246)

1. In a microwave-safe dish, combine the cacao butter and coconut oil. Microwave for 1 minute. Stir and then microwave in 30-second increments until melted completely.

2. Whisk in the cacao powder and sweetener, adjusting the sweetness to your liking.

3. Arrange 12 silicone or parchment paper muffin cups on a baking sheet. Pour ½ tablespoon of the melted chocolate mixture into the bottom of each muffin cup. Place in the freezer for 10 minutes.

4. Remove from the freezer and top each muffin cup with ½ tablespoon of nut butter and press down to evenly cover the bottom chocolate layer. Freeze for another 10 minutes.

5. Remove from the freezer and top with ½ tablespoon of the melted chocolate mixture. Freeze for another 10 minutes or until solid.

6. Store in the freezer for up to 3 months.

INGREDIENT TIP: Replace the hazelnut butter with another low-carb nut butter of choice or coconut butter/manna.

PER SERVING (1 nut butter cup)

Calories: 181; Total Fat: 19g; Protein: 1g; Total Carbs: 1.5g; Fiber: 1g; Net Carbs: 0.5g

FUDGY KETO BROWNIES

MAKES 16 BROWNIES | PREP TIME: 20 MINUTES | COOK TIME: 20 MINUTES

PALEO/DAIRY-FREE OPTION · BULK PREP

Brownies were a staple in my household growing up. These brownies are extremely moist, super chocolaty, and go perfectly with a glass of unsweetened coconut milk.

Butter or coconut oil, for greasing

1 cup chocolate collagen powder
  (I use Perfect Keto)

½ cup almond flour

¼ cup unsweetened cacao/
  cocoa powder

½ teaspoon baking soda

¼ teaspoon sea salt

6 tablespoons granulated sweetener
  such as Swerve

⅓ cup smooth almond butter
  (or nut butter of choice)

2 tablespoons butter, melted

2 eggs

1 teaspoon vanilla extract

½ teaspoon nondairy milk (hemp,
  almond, macadamia, coconut)

3 tablespoons brewed coffee, cold, or
  1 tablespoon instant coffee (optional)

⅛ cup Lily's chocolate chips (optional)

1. Preheat the oven to 350°F. Grease an 8-inch square baking dish with butter or coconut oil.

2. In a medium bowl, whisk together the collagen powder, almond flour, cacao powder, baking soda, salt, and sweetener.

3. In a small microwave-safe bowl, combine the almond butter and butter. Microwave for 10 to 15 seconds until melted.

4. Add the butter mixture, eggs, vanilla, nondairy milk, and coffee (if using) to the dry ingredients and mix until smooth.

5. Pour the batter into the prepared baking dish and spread evenly. Top with the chocolate chips (if using).

6. Bake for 18 to 20 minutes or until a knife inserted in the center comes out clean.

INGREDIENT TIP: You can use unflavored collagen powder but will need to add an additional ¼ cup of cacao/cocoa powder.

MAKE IT PALEO/DAIRY-FREE: Replace the butter with coconut oil.

PER SERVING (1 brownie)

Calories: 112; Total Fat: 8g; Protein: 6g; Total Carbs: 4g; Fiber: 2g; Net Carbs: 2g

COCONUT–WHITE CHOCOLATE FUDGE

MAKES 16 SQUARES | PREP TIME: 10 MINUTES, PLUS OVERNIGHT TO CHILL

EGG-FREE · NUT-FREE · PALEO/DAIRY-FREE · VEGETARIAN · BULK PREP

The number of ingredients that come from a coconut is pretty crazy. Coconut water, milk, cream, butter, oil, vinegar, aminos, flakes, and the list goes on. If I had to choose my favorite coconut ingredient, it would definitely be coconut butter/manna. I could live off this stuff (see note below for more info). This is my take on keto white chocolate fudge!

Coconut oil for greasing

1 cup full-fat unsweetened coconut milk

4 ounces unsweetened cacao/cocoa butter, chopped

½ cup coconut butter/manna

⅓ cup vanilla-flavored collagen powder

1 teaspoon vanilla extract

¼ teaspoon sea salt

⅛ teaspoon ground cinnamon (optional)

½ teaspoon sweetener of choice (optional)

1. Grease an 8-inch square pan with oil and then line it with a piece of parchment paper, pressing down so that it sticks and evenly covers the pan.

2. In a medium saucepan over low heat, melt together the coconut milk, cacao butter, and coconut butter, stirring occasionally, until smooth. Remove from the heat and whisk in the collagen powder, vanilla, salt, and cinnamon (if using). Taste the mixture and then add the sweetener (if using), adjusting the sweetness to your liking.

3. Pour the mixture into the prepared pan and spread evenly. Refrigerate overnight.

4. Cut into 16 squares and store in an airtight container in the refrigerator for up to 2 weeks.

INGREDIENT TIP: Don't confuse coconut butter (also known as coconut manna) for coconut oil. They are very different. Coconut oil is the oil extracted from coconut meat while coconut butter is the actual flesh of the coconut meat ground into a paste or butter. It can be found in most grocery stores or sold online. Sometimes the oil and butter separate in the jar and you may need to microwave it for 30 to 40 seconds or until melted. Then mix well to combine.

PER SERVING (1 square)

Calories: 148; Total Fat: 15g; Protein: 2g; Total Carbs: 2g; Fiber: 1g; Net Carbs: 1g

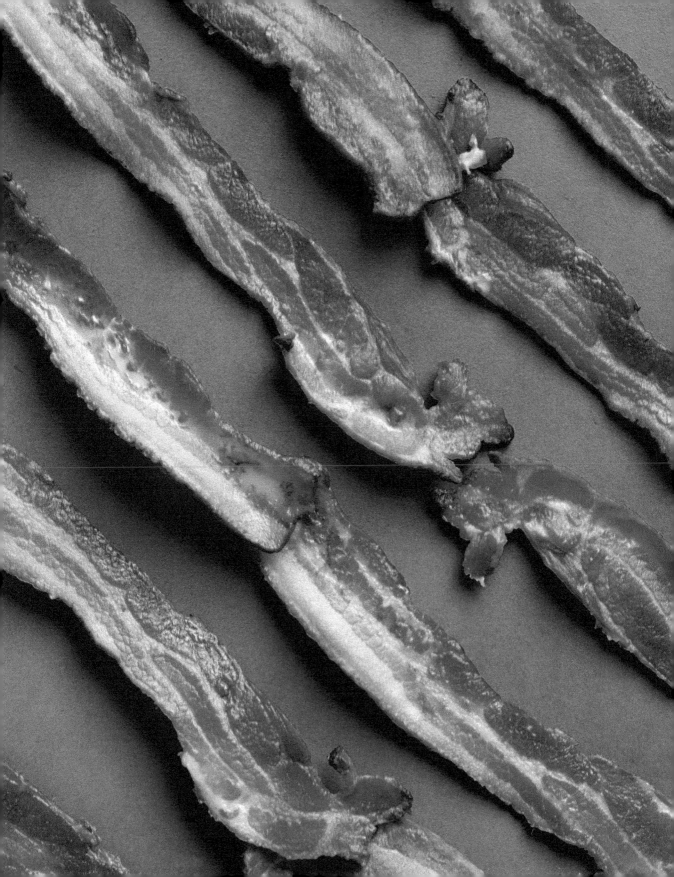

MEASUREMENT CONVERSIONS

Volume Equivalents (Liquid)

STANDARD	US STANDARD (OUNCES)	METRIC (APPROXIMATE)
2 tablespoons	1 fl. oz.	30 mL
¼ cup	2 fl. oz.	60 mL
½ cup	4 fl. oz.	120 mL
1 cup	8 fl. oz.	240 mL
1½ cups	12 fl. oz.	355 mL
2 cups or 1 pint	16 fl. oz.	475 mL
4 cups or 1 quart	32 fl. oz.	1 L
1 gallon	128 fl. oz.	4 L

Oven Temperatures

FAHRENHEIT (F)	CELSIUS (C) (APPROXIMATE)
250°	120°
300°	150°
325°	165°
350°	180°
375°	190°
400°	200°
425°	220°
450°	230°

Volume Equivalents (Dry)

STANDARD	METRIC (APPROXIMATE)
⅛ teaspoon	0.5 mL
¼ teaspoon	1 mL
½ teaspoon	2 mL
¾ teaspoon	4 mL
1 teaspoon	5 mL
1 tablespoon	15 mL
¼ cup	59 mL
⅓ cup	79 mL
½ cup	118 mL
⅔ cup	156 mL
¾ cup	177 mL
1 cup	235 mL
2 cups or 1 pint	475 mL
3 cups	700 mL
4 cups or 1 quart	1 L

Weight Equivalents

STANDARD	METRIC (APPROXIMATE)
½ ounce	15 g
1 ounce	30 g
2 ounces	60 g
4 ounces	115 g
8 ounces	225 g
12 ounces	340 g
16 ounces or 1 pound	455 g

RESOURCES

WEBSITES AND BLOGS

Rachel Gregory, KillinItKeto.com

Amanda C. Hughes, WickedStuffed.com

Dr. Anthony Gustin, DrAnthonyGustin.com

Dr. Bret Scher, LowCarbCardiologist.com

Dr. Brian Lenzkes, LowCarbAdvisor.com

Dr. Jacob Wilson, TheASPI.com

Dr. Ryan Lowery, Ketogenic.com

Brian Williamson and Danny Vega, Ketovangelist.com

Chris Irvin, TheKetologist.com

Danny and Maura Vega, FatFueled.family

Dave Feldman, CholesterolCode.com

Doug Reynolds and Pam Devine, LowCarbUSA.org

Drew Manning, Fit2Fat2Fit.com

Jason Wittrock, JasonWittrock.com

Jeff Kotterman, TriSystem.network/low-carb-options

Jen Fisch, KetoInTheCity.com

Jimmy Moore, LivinLaVidaLowCarb.com

Keto Connect, KetoConnect.net

Ketogains, Ketogains.com

Leanne Vogel, HealthfulPursuit.com

Robert Sikes and Crystal Love, KetoSavage.com

ONLINE TOOLS AND APPS

Keto-Friendly Products
KillinItKeto.com/keto-alternatives—Alternatives Access to keto-friendly brands and products mentioned throughout this book with discounts included for each.

Keto Macro Calculators
Keto-Calculator.ankerl.com
MariaMindBodyHealth.com/keto-calculator
PerfectKeto.com/keto-macro-calculator

Body Fat Calculator
US Navy Body Fat Calculator — fitness.bizcalcs.com/Calculator
.asp?Calc=Body-Fat-Navy

Apps
Senza — A completely free, keto-specific meal tracking and learning app that includes a built-in macro calculator, keto-specific food tracking, daily recipes and tips, and much more.

REFERENCES

Bueno, Nassib, Ingrid Vieira de Melo, Suzana Lima de Oliveira, Terezinha da Rocha Ataide. "Very-Low-Carbohydrate Ketogenic Diet v. Low-Fat Diet for Long-Term Weight Loss: A Meta-Analysis of Randomised Controlled Trials." *British Journal of Nutrition* 110, no. 7 (October 2013): 1178–87. doi:10.1017 /S0007114513000548.

Dehghan, Mahshid et al. "Associations of Fats and Carbohydrate Intake with Cardiovascular Disease and Mortality in 18 Countries from Five Continents (PURE): A Prospective Cohort Study." *The Lancet* 390, no. 10107 (November 2017): 2050–62. doi:10.1016/S0140-6736(17)32252-3.

Emmerich, Maria, and Craig Emmerich. *Keto.* Victory Belt Publishing, 2018.

Gedgaudas, Nora. *Primal Fat Burner.* New York: Atria Books, 2017.

Gregory, Rachel, Hasan Hamdan, Danielle Torisky, Jeremy Akers. "A Low-Carbohydrate Ketogenic Diet Combined with 6-Weeks of Crossfit Training Improves Body Composition and Performance." *International Journal of Sports and Exercise Medicine* 3, no. 2 (March 2017) doi:10.23937/2469-5718/1510054.

Kearns, Cristin, Laura Schmidt, and Stanton Glantz. "Sugar Industry and Coronary Heart Disease Research: A Historical Analysis of Internal Industry Documents." *Journal of the American Medical Association* 176, no. 11 (November 2016): 1680–85. doi:10.1001/jamainternmed.2016.5394.

Mercola, Dr. Joseph. *Fat For Fuel.* California: Hay House, Inc., 2017.

National Institute of Diabetes and Digestive and Kidney Diseases. "Overweight and Obesity Statistics." Accessed March 5, 2018. www.niddk.nih.gov/health -information/health-statistics/overweight-obesity.

Paoli, Antonio, Adriano Rubini, Jeff Volek, Keith Grimaldi. "Beyond Weight Loss: A Review of the Therapeutic Uses of Very-Low-Carbohydrate (Ketogenic) Diets." *European Journal of Clinical Nutrition* 67, no. 8 (June 2013): 789–96. doi:10.1038 /ejcn.2013.116.

Reaven, Gerald. "Pathophysiology of Insulin Resistance in Human Disease." *Physiological Reviews* 75, no. 3 (July 1995): 473–86. doi:10.1152/physrev .1995.75.3.473.

United States Department of Agriculture. "Dietary Guidelines." Accessed March 10, 2018. www.choosemyplate.gov/dietary-guidelines.

Volek, Jeff, and Stephen Phinney. *The Art and Science of Low Carbohydrate Living.* Beyond Obesity LLC, 2011.

———. *The Art and Science of Low Carbohydrate Performance.* Beyond Obesity LLC, 2012.

Way, Kimberley, Daniel Hackett, Michael Baker, Nathan Johnson. "The Effect of Regular Exercise on Insulin Sensitivity in Type 2 Diabetes Mellitus: A Systematic Review and Meta-Analysis." *Diabetes & Metabolism Journal* 40, no. 4 (August 2016): 253–271. doi:10.4093/dmj.2016.40.4.253.

Wilson, Jacob, and Ryan Lowery. *The Ketogenic Bible: The Authoritative Guide to Ketosis.* Victory Belt Publishing, 2017.

RECIPE INDEX

INDEX

ACKNOWLEDGMENTS

I'd like to thank my family and friends who have encouraged me to follow my passion and who have helped make this book possible. To my parents, Robin and Jim, my sister, Jenna, and my partner in crime, Alex, thank you for always being there for me and especially for supporting me throughout this book-writing and recipe-testing process. To all my clients and other friends who have tested my recipes and given amazing feedback and suggestions, you are amazing and I am so grateful to have you in my life.

I'd also like to give a huge shout-out to all of my friends and colleagues within the keto community. You all are rock stars and I am so fortunate to be able to work with amazing, extremely passionate people who strive to make this world a healthier place. I'm excited to continue making new relationships within this community and I can't wait to see what the future holds for us all!

ABOUT THE AUTHORS

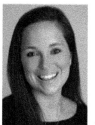

Rachel Gregory, MS, CNS, ATC, CSCS, is a board-certified nutrition specialist, athletic trainer, and strength and conditioning coach. She received her master's degree in nutrition and exercise physiology from James Madison University and bachelor's degree in sports medicine from the University of Miami.

Rachel has vast knowledge on the science and application of the ketogenic diet for weight loss, performance, and overall health. She completed the *first* human clinical trial looking at the effects of the ketogenic diet in CrossFit athletes, which was published in the *International Journal of Sports and Exercise Medicine*. Rachel has presented her research at national conferences and works closely with several doctors and scientists specializing in the low-carbohydrate, ketogenic lifestyle.

Rachel is the **founder and CEO of Killin It Keto, LLC** and creator of the **21-Day Keto Challenge**. She has worked with a variety of individuals throughout her career that include Division I collegiate athletes, WNBA stars, and some of the top bodybuilders in the world. She has a passion for educating those interested in optimizing their physical and mental well-being while improving long-term health goals. Find her at KillinItKeto.com.

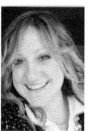

Amanda C. Hughes is a ketogenic chef based in New England with nearly a decade of experience in developing and cooking popular low-carb and Paleo recipes. She is the author of the best-selling *Wicked Good Ketogenic Diet Cookbook*. Her ketogenic food adventure blog, WickedStuffed.com, has been described as "life-saving," "hilarious," "delicious," and "nonsense free" by the millions of keto-loving home chefs who read her blog and cook her recipes.

Sunday
Jalapeño poppers
nutbread cookies

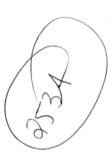

9 781623 159320